# Controlled Substance Risk Mitigation in the Dental Setting

*Editors*

RONALD J. KULICH
DAVID A. KEITH
MICHAEL E. SCHATMAN

# DENTAL CLINICS OF NORTH AMERICA

www.dental.theclinics.com

July 2020 • Volume 64 • Number 3

**ELSEVIER**

1600 John F. Kennedy Boulevard • Suite 1800 • Philadelphia, Pennsylvania, 19103-2899

http://www.dental.theclinics.com

**DENTAL CLINICS OF NORTH AMERICA Volume 64, Number 3**
**July 2020 ISSN 0011-8532, ISBN: 978-0-323-76109-3**

Editor: John Vassallo; j.vassallo@elsevier.com
Developmental Editor: Laura Fisher

*Dental Clinics of North America* (ISSN 0011-8532) is published quarterly by Elsevier Inc., 360 Park Avenue South, New York, NY 10010-1710. Months of issue are January, April, July, and October. Business and Editorial Offices: 1600 John F. Kennedy Boulevard, Suite 1800, Philadelphia, PA 19103-2899. Periodicals postage paid at New York, NY and additional mailing offices. Subscription prices are $304.00 per year (domestic individuals), $633.00 per year (domestic institutions), $100.00 per year (domestic students/residents), $366.00 per year (Canadian individuals), $821.00 per year (Canadian institutions), $100.00 per year (Canadian students/residents) $424.00 per year (international individuals), $821.00 per year (international institutions), and $200.00 per year (international students/residents). International air speed delivery is included in all *Clinics* subscription prices. All prices are subject to change without notice. **POSTMASTER:** Send address changes to *Dental Clinics of North America*, Elsevier Health Sciences Division, Subscription Customer Service, 3251 Riverport Lane, Maryland Heights, MO 63043. **Customer Service (orders, claims, online, change of address): Elsevier Health Sciences Division, Subscription Customer Service, 3251 Riverport Lane, Maryland Heights, MO 63043. Tel: 1-800-654-2452 (U.S. and Canada). Fax: 314-447-8029. E-mail: journalscustomerservice-usa@elsevier.com (for print support); journalsonlinesupport-usa@elsevier. com (for online support).**

*Reprints.* For copies of 100 or more, of articles in this publication, please contact the Commercial Reprints Department, Elsevier Inc., 360 Park Avenue South, New York, NY 10010-1710. Tel.: 212-633-3874; Fax: 212-633-3820; E-mail: reprints@elsevier.com.

The *Dental Clinics of North America* is covered in *MEDLINE/PubMed (Index Medicus), Current Contents/Clinical Medicine, ISI/BIOMED* and *Clinahl*.

# Contributors

## EDITORS

**RONALD J. KULICH, PhD**
Professor, Department of Diagnostic Sciences, Tufts University School of Dental Medicine; Lecturer, Department of Anesthesia, Critical Care and Pain Medicine, Massachusetts General Hospital, Harvard Medical School, Boston, Massachusetts, USA

**DAVID A. KEITH, BDS, FDSRCS, DMD**
Visiting Oral and Maxillofacial Surgeon, Massachusetts General Hospital, Professor, Oral and Maxillofacial Surgery, Harvard School of Dental Medicine, Boston, Massachusetts, USA

**MICHAEL E. SCHATMAN, PhD**
Adjunct Associate, Department of Diagnostic Sciences, Tufts University School of Dental Medicine, Adjunct Clinical Assistant Professor, Department of Public Health and Community Medicine, Tufts University School of Medicine, Boston, Massachusetts, USA

## AUTHORS

**DONAVON KHOSROW K. ARONI, DMD, MS**
Assistant Professor, Division of Craniofacial Pain and Headache, Tufts University School of Dental Medicine, Boston, Massachusetts, USA

**ANTJE M. BARREVELD, MD**
Assistant Professor, Department of Anesthesiology, Tufts University School of Medicine, Boston, Massachusetts, USA; Medical Director, Pain Management Services, Director of Education and Outreach, Substance Use Services, Newton-Wellesley Hospital, Newton, Massachusetts, USA

**SHUCHI DHADWAL, DMD**
Assistant Professor, Director of the Craniofacial Pain Center, Department of Diagnostic Sciences, Tufts University School of Dental Medicine, Boston, Massachusetts, USA

**MATTHEW FORTINO, MA**
Clinical Intern, Department of Diagnostic Sciences, Tufts University School of Dental Medicine, Research Associate, Department of Anesthesia, Critical Care and Pain Medicine, Harvard Medical School, Massachusetts General Hospital, Boston, Massachusetts, USA; Doctoral Student, William James College, Newton, Massachusetts, USA

**HUDSON FRANCA, MD**
Resident in Internal Medicine, Universidad Iberoamericana, Santo Domingo, Dominican Republic; Tufts University School of Dental Medicine, Boston, Massachusetts, USA

**RICHARD S. HAROLD, DMD, JD**
Associate Professor, Department of Comprehensive Care, Tufts University School of Dental Medicine, Boston, Massachusetts, USA

**MARÍA F. HERNÁNDEZ-NUÑO DE LA ROSA , DDS, MS**
Dental Sleep Medicine Fellow, Craniofacial Pain and Sleep Center, Department of Diagnostic Sciences, Tufts University School of Dental Medicine, Boston, Massachusetts, USA

**VANAK HUOT, RDH, MPH**
Department of Clinical Affairs, Tufts University School of Dental Medicine, Boston, Massachusetts, USA

**JOSHUA A. KAUFMAN, MD**
Department of Psychiatry, Columbia University, New York State Psychiatric Institute, New York, New York, USA

**DAVID A. KEITH, BDS, FDSRCS, DMD**
Visiting Oral and Maxillofacial Surgeon, Massachusetts General Hospital, Professor, Oral and Maxillofacial Surgery, Harvard School of Dental Medicine, Boston, Massachusetts, USA

**SHEHRYAR NASIR KHAWAJA, BDS, MSc**
Diplomat, American Board of Orofacial Pain; Consultant, Orofacial Pain Medicine, Department of Internal Medicine, Shaukat Khanum Memorial Cancer Hospital and Research Centre, Lahore, Punjab, Pakistan

**RONALD J. KULICH, PhD**
Professor, Department of Diagnostic Sciences, Tufts University School of Dental Medicine; Lecturer, Department of Anesthesia, Critical Care and Pain Medicine, Massachusetts General Hospital, Harvard Medical School, Boston, Massachusetts, USA

**JENNIFER MAGEE, DMD, MPH**
Director, MGH Dental Group – Danvers, Assistant in Dentistry, Department of Oral Surgery, Instructor, Harvard School of Dental Medicine, Boston, Massachusetts, USA

**BRITTA E. MAGNUSON, DMD**
Assistant Professor, Department of Diagnostic Sciences, Tufts University School of Dental Medicine, Boston, Massachusetts, USA

**PRIYANKA MONGA, DDS**
Orofacial Pain Resident, Department of Diagnostic Sciences, Tufts University School of Dental Medicine, Boston, Massachusetts, USA

**ELLEN PATTERSON, MD**
Assistant Professor, Director of Behavioral Science Education, Department of Comprehensive Care, Tufts University School of Dental Medicine, Boston, Massachusetts, USA

**MICHAEL E. SCHATMAN, PhD**
Adjunct Associate, Department of Diagnostic Sciences, Tufts University School of Dental Medicine, Adjunct Clinical Assistant Professor, Department of Public Health and Community Medicine, Tufts University School of Medicine, Boston, Massachusetts, USA

**STEVEN JOHN SCRIVANI, DDS, DMSc**
Former Professor, Department of Diagnostic Sciences, Craniofacial Pain Center, Tufts University School of Dental Medicine, Adjunct Visiting Professor, Pain Research, Education and Policy Program, Department of Public Health and Community Medicine, Tufts University School of Medicine, Boston, Massachusetts, USA

**HANNAH SHAPIRO**
Department of Biopsychology, Tufts University, Medford, Massachusetts, USA

**HUW F. THOMAS, BDS, MS, PhD**
Professor of Pediatric Dentistry, Tufts University School of Dental Medicine, Boston, Massachusetts, USA

**RICHARD W. VALACHOVIC, DMD, MPH**
President emeritus, American Dental Education Association, Visiting Scholar, New York University College of Dentistry, New York, New York, USA

**ALEXIS A. VASCIANNIE**
Department of Diagnostic Sciences, Tufts University School of Dental Medicine, Boston, Massachusetts, USA

**ARCHANA VISWANATH, BDS, MS**
Assistant Professor and Director of Clinical Research, Departments of Oral and Maxillofacial Surgery, and Diagnostic Sciences, Tufts University School of Dental Medicine, Boston, Massachusetts, USA

# Contents

**Preface** xi

Ronald J. Kulich, David A. Keith, and Michael E. Schatman

**Introduction** xv

Richard W. Valachovic

**Dentistry's Role in Assessing and Managing Controlled Substance Risk: Historical
Overview, Current Barriers, and Working Toward Best Practices** 491

Shuchi Dhadwal, Ronald J. Kulich, Priyanka Monga, and Michael E. Schatman

Dentistry is in a unique position among the health care professions to assess and manage the patient with controlled substance risk. The concern over opioid risk is not new, and historically dentists have had to balance the critical need for adequate pain care with the importance of recognizing the consequences of using controlled substances for their patients. Barriers for providing adequate patient assessment and management may be greater in dentistry than other health care fields, although these barriers can be recognized and overcome. Collaboration with co-treating providers will improve patient outcomes and reduce patient risk.

**Patient Interviewing Strategies to Recognize Substance Use, Misuse, and Abuse in
the Dental Setting** 503

Michael E. Schatman, Ellen Patterson, and Hannah Shapiro

Brief and effective clinical interviewing is critical for identifying patient risk factors, including those associated with substance use. Dental practitioners may perceive identifying patient substance misuse and abuse as a complex undertaking or may consider this clinical assessment beyond the scope of their training and practice. This article describes interviewing strategies that will help dental providers communicate effectively and empathically with their patients to collect relevant clinical information related to substance use, misuse, and abuse and provide better care for their patients.

**Special Screening Resources: Strategies to Identify Substance Use Disorders,
Including Opioid Misuse and Abuse** 513

David A. Keith and María F. Hernández-Nuño de la Rosa

The prescription drug crisis has affected all sectors of the population, and so it is inevitable that dentists will increasingly see at-risk patients or those with substance use disorders in the course of their professional activities. Recognizing these patients and the special needs that they may have is now part of the standard of care for the profession. Screening for substance misuse involves a thorough history and review of the patient's medical record and, as appropriate, reviewing prior records and use of available screening tools.

**Managing Acute Dental Pain: Principles for Rational Prescribing and Alternatives to Opioid Therapy**                                                                    525

Shehryar Nasir Khawaja and Steven John Scrivani

> Pharmacotherapy forms an integral part of acute dental pain management. In a majority of cases, safe and effective management of acute dental pain can be accomplished with a non-opioid medication regimen. Nonetheless, in certain circumstances use of opioid medications may be needed. Furthermore, there are various pain management regimens, such as pre-emptive analgesia, post-procedural cold compression, use of long acting anesthetic, and compound drug therapy that can improve the efficacy of analgesics to achieve a desired therapeutic response without compromising patient safety.

**Comorbid Conditions in Relation to Controlled Substance Abuse**                    535

Matthew Fortino, Ronald J. Kulich, Joshua A. Kaufman, and Hudson Franca

> Dental patients who experience comorbid psychiatric and medical conditions present an elevated risk of medication misuse, abuse, substance use disorders, and overdose. The authors review the role of notable comorbidities in predicting the development of substance use disorder, including medical, psychiatric, and other psychosocial factors that can be assessed in general dental practice. Psychiatric disorders commonly cooccur with substance abuse, and these typically include anxiety disorders, mood disorders (major depression, bipolar), posttraumatic stress, as well as sleep and eating disorders. Medical disorders commonly found to be present with substance use disorders are also reviewed, including common cardiovascular and pulmonary disorders.

**Assessment and Management of the High-Risk Dental Patient with Active Substance Use Disorder**                                                                    547

Archana Viswanath, Antje M. Barreveld, and Matthew Fortino

> Every dentist cares for patients with a history of substance use disorder (SUD), regardless of a patient's socioeconomic status, education, or ethnicity. SUD is a global epidemic, with approximately 8% of the general US population meeting diagnostic criteria for a SUD and more than 20% of the global population experiencing a SUD. The importance of understanding how to identify substance use, manage patients with a SUD, and offer appropriate referral is essential for all dental professionals. In 2005, the American Dental Association published, "Statement on Provision of Dental Treatment for Patients with Substance Use Disorders."

**Brief Motivational Interventions: Strategies for Successful Management of Complex, Nonadherent Dental Patients**                                                    559

Michael E. Schatman, Hannah Shapiro, María F. Hernández-Nuño de la Rosa, and Vanak Huot

> Motivational interviewing (MI) is an evidence-based approach to resolving patient ambivalence to change. MI techniques can be effectively used by dentists in assessing and managing substance use risk and may add minimal time to the patient interview. Although MI's greatest utility has been in the area of improving general oral hygiene in order to reduce caries and

other preventable conditions, its use in addressing controlled substance risk is well established in other health care disciplines. These techniques do not require special training in mental health assessment and can be effectively used by dentists and dental hygienists.

## Interprofessional Collaboration in the Assessment and Management of Substance Use Risk

571

Ronald J. Kulich, David A. Keith, Alexis A. Vasciannie, and Huw F. Thomas

Substance use disorder assessment strategies are increasingly being employed by dentistry, while adequate evaluation requires reaching out to other cotreating providers and collaborating on patient care. The field of dentistry has a range of barriers often not experienced in other professions, including limitations on e-record communication and clinical practice setting often isolated from the patient's general medical care. Barriers can be overcome if the dentist facilitates communication.

## Special High-Risk Populations in Dentistry: The Adolescent Patient, the Elderly Patient, and the Woman of Childbearing Age

585

Jennifer Magee, Britta E. Magnuson, and Donavon Khosrow K. Aroni

Comprehensive and compassionate treatment of vulnerable patients is an important service to the community, although dental treatment of special populations can represent a challenge. The dental provider must be able to recognize the issues surrounding substance use and abuse, coordinate care with medical providers, and build a trusting provider–patient relationship to achieve success. Open conversations regarding expectations of pain, and the risks, benefits, and alternatives to opioids are important aspects of the best care of these patients.

## Opioid Prescribing in Dental Practice: Managing Liability Risks

597

David A. Keith, Ronald J. Kulich, Alexis A. Vasciannie, and Richard S. Harold

Dentistry should be proud of its history of providing responsible pain relief, as well as becoming more cautious in prescribing opioid medications when other safer pharmacologic options exist. Our training directs us to first eliminate the source of dental pain and prescribe analgesics only as adjunctive relief. Prescriptions must be written for a legitimate dental purpose and for a patient of record. Through self-regulation, the dental profession must continue to establish pain management guidelines based on scientific evidence and clinical experience to avoid further regulatory action restricting our prescribing privileges, which remain one of our most powerful therapeutic tools.

# DENTAL CLINICS OF NORTH AMERICA

**FORTHCOMING ISSUES**

*October 2020*
**The Journey to Excellence in Esthetic Dentistry**
Yair Y. Whiteman and David J. Wagner, *Editors*

*January 2021*
**Implant Surgery Update for the General Practitioner**
Harry Dym, *Editor*

*April 2021*
**Geriatric Dental Medicine**
Joseph M. Calabrese and Michelle Henshaw, *Editors*

**RECENT ISSUES**

*April 2020*
**Surgical and Medical Management of Common Oral Problems**
Harry Dym, *Editor*

*January 2020*
**Oral Diseases for the General Dentist**
Arvind Babu Rajendra Santosh and Orrett E. Ogle, *Editors*

*October 2019*
**Caries Management**
Sandra Guzmán-Armstrong, Margherita Fontana, Marcelle M. Nascimento, and Andrea G. Ferreira Zandona, *Editors*

**SERIES OF RELATED INTEREST**

*Atlas of the Oral and Maxillofacial Surgery Clinics*
http://www.oralmaxsurgeryatlas.theclinics.com

*Oral and Maxillofacial Surgery Clinics*
http://www.oralmaxsurgery.theclinics.com

# Preface

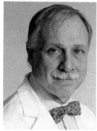 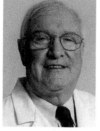 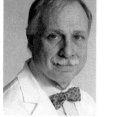

Ronald J. Kulich, PhD    David A. Keith, BDS, FDSRCS, DMD    Michael E. Schatman, PhD

*Editors*

Dentists have been on the forefront of pain management for well over 4000 years.[1] In fact, it was a dentist, William Morton, who pioneered the first public demonstration of anesthesia at Massachusetts General Hospital in 1843, an event that made possible the development of Surgery as we know it today. In the years that followed, a range of oral analgesics also was developed as a mainstay of acute pain management in dental care. With all of these efforts, the late nineteenth century brought a recognition that prescribed opioids for pain could pose addiction-related risks.[2] By the late twentieth century, following the lead of other health care specialty groups, dentists were encouraged to aggressively prescribe opioids for acute pain, and they remained the second highest-volume prescriber group of any specialty for a number of years. Concurrent with these historical events, the high prevalence of substance use disorders persisted, with particular increased risks for the misuse and abuse of opioids during the initial decade of this millennium. Throughout their long histories of providing effective care for acute pain, dentists have remained a health care subspecialty that maintained close relationships with their patients, often seeing them more often than their physician counterparts. With this history, the role and responsibilities of dentists continued to expand, and the concept of "interprofessional" collaboration has seen increased attention at all levels of dental school training. Indeed, the base rates in the population suggest that dentists will see patients who are at risk for substance misuse and abuse on a daily basis, a fact that necessitates a close interaction with other providers. With dentistry's expanding role, there remains a unique opportunity to identify and assess patients who are at risk for substance use disorders, as well as provide effective care that leads to recovery where substance abuse may be present.

Dent Clin N Am 64 (2020) xi–xiii
https://doi.org/10.1016/j.cden.2020.04.001
0011-8532/20/© 2020 Published by Elsevier Inc.

In his introduction to the issue, Dr Valachovic underscores the important role of dentistry in mitigating substance use risk, but also highlights the role of the dental hygienist as an active member of the team. Dr Dhadwal and associates discuss strategies for achieving best practices in substance use disorder assessment and management, while recognizing current barriers specific to the field of dentistry. Underscoring the importance of managing acute pain in the context of the patient with substance use risk, Drs Khawaja and Scrivani outline current standard-of-care approaches with respect to the pharmacologic management of acute pain. Dr Schatman and his colleagues review practical interviewing strategies for dental patients with the most complex substance use risk presentations and offer a useful template for implementing Motivational Interviewing strategies in dental settings in another article. Kulich and his coauthors address the importance of interprofessional care in dentistry, barriers to such care, and strategies for advancing cross-disciplinary cooperation. Use of validated measures remains a mainstay of assessment, and Drs Keith and colleagues review validated measures for assessing the patient with complex substance use conditions, offering special attention to utilizing state prescription drug monitoring programs. Fortino and co-authors discuss the common psychiatric and medical comorbidities concomitant to a diagnosis of substance use disorder and offer practical assessment and management strategies for the non–mental health provider. Drawing from the substance use treatment literature, Dr Viswanath's and Dr Magee's articles address active substance-abusing patients as well as the special populations that have been seriously impacted by substance use disorders. Populations discussed include adolescents, women of child-bearing age, the elderly, and individuals who have experienced major emotional or physical trauma. Finally, Dr Keith and his colleagues review the medicolegal issues surrounding the treatment and management of this complex population, offering strategies for minimizing risks for providers.

We were fortunate to bring together the authors of this project from across the United States, with the mission of preparing additional materials intended for virtual teaching of the topics outlined in this series. We intend this to act as a companion text for a series of Web-based training modules on controlled substance risk mitigation currently in development. The latter has been undertaken as a project currently being funded through a grant from the Coverys Community Healthcare Foundation.

Ronald J. Kulich, PhD
Department of Diagnostic Sciences
Tufts University School of Dental Medicine
Department of Anesthesia
Critical Care and Pain Medicine
Harvard Medical School
Massachusetts General Hospital
1 Kneeland Street
Boston, MA 02111, USA

David A. Keith, BDS, FDSRCS, DMD
Massachusetts General Hospital
Oral and Maxillofacial Surgery
Harvard School of Dental Medicine
Warren 1201, Fruit Street
Boston, MA 02114, USA

Michael E. Schatman, PhD
Department of Diagnostic Sciences
Tufts University School of Dental Medicine
Department of Public Health and
Community Medicine
Tufts University School of Medicine
1 Kneeland Street
Boston, MA 02111, USA

*E-mail addresses:*
rkulich@mgh.harvard.edu (R.J. Kulich)
DKeith@partners.org (D.A. Keith)
Michael.schatman@tufts.edu (M.E. Schatman)

**REFERENCES**

1. Escohotado A. The general history of drugs, vol. 1. Valparaiso (Chile): Graffiti Militante Press; 2010 [Robinette GW, Trans].
2. Kulich R, Loeser JD. The business of pain medicine: the present mirrors antiquity. Pain Med 2011;12(7):1063–75.

# Introduction

Dental pain is real, and most dentists in practice were taught that the most effective way to alleviate severe pain was with opioid painkillers. That's what I was taught during my dental school experience and my residency in pediatric dentistry. During the early part of my career in dental education, I served as Dean for Clinical Affairs at the dental schools at Harvard University and the University of Connecticut. Students and residents faced with patients who presented complaining of pain were eager to address their symptoms, and opioids were often prescribed for them. The medications worked well; there was little evidence of nonprescription alternatives, and there was not a full appreciation of the concerns about patients misusing or abusing these medications. Later in my career, I was appointed the CEO of what is now the American Dental Education Association headquartered in Washington, DC. This was during the initial phases of the opioid epidemic in the 1990s, and I witnessed firsthand how compelling the scourge of the epidemic was as it began to run its course throughout the nation. Many were surprised to learn that dentists were among the main prescribers of opioids, especially for adolescents and young adults.[1] We know that we in dentistry contributed to the onset of the epidemic, and we now need to take an active role in resolving it. A key component in that effort is to mitigate the risks of misuse and abuse in the dental setting.

Lives are at stake. It is estimated that 130 Americans die each day from an opioid overdose.[2] The number of opioids prescribed by dentists has decreased substantially over the past 2 decades, but we should continue to do all that we can as dental professionals to address the opioid epidemic in every way possible.[3]

This issue of *Dental Clinics of North America* is a significant contribution to that goal. It is authored by a team comprised mostly of Boston-based clinicians and researchers who have worked together for years on developing evidence-based strategies to address the problem, particularly those strategies that assist clinicians in identifying and working with patients at risk for misuse or abuse of prescription medications. Much of the research into the origins of the misuse and abuse of opioid medications and strategies to deal with these complex patients that has evolved over the past 2 decades has been conducted by these authors. As a result, this issue is remarkably current in providing practitioners with an understanding of the breadth of the issues as well as the strategies required to mitigate risk. They worked with the governor of Massachusetts to develop a collaboration between the 3 dental schools in the state that produced core competencies for the prevention and management of prescription drug abuse.[4] Massachusetts developed a Drug Prescription Monitoring Program that collects dispensing information on controlled substances to help prescribers deter drug diversion and assess whether patients might be at risk for drug abuse. These practices are being disseminated throughout other states as well.

Those of us in dentistry have always had to deal with an unfortunate public perception of an association with pain. In dealing with policymakers in Washington and other health professionals in general, I have found it worthwhile to highlight data that reflect the dental status of the US population and the reasons we are often confronted with patients in distress. About 20% of children aged 5 to 11 years and about 13% of

Dent Clin N Am 64 (2020) xv–xvii
https://doi.org/10.1016/j.cden.2020.04.002
0011-8532/20/© 2020 Published by Elsevier Inc.

adolescents have at least 1 untreated tooth with dental caries.[5] Nearly half of adults show signs of periodontal disease.[6] There are about 3.5 million people each year who have third-molar extractions.[7] Dentists need to have an armamentarium of medications to address those patients in pain; the issue is developing the strategies to provide the appropriate drugs to the appropriate patients for the appropriate amount of time while reducing opportunities for drug misuse or abuse. This issue provides an abundance of scientifically based information and protocols to help the clinician make these decisions.

Much has been done recently to address the ability of current dental students and residents to deal with patients who present in acute pain. The competencies for safe prescribing that were developed with the dental schools in Massachusetts are a phenomenal start and are being shared throughout the country. The Commission on Dental Accreditation has revised its standards to emphasize dental students' competencies in local anesthesia, pain, and anxiety control in the prescription practices on substance abuse disorders. Dental students are being taught to use electronic health records and prescription drug monitoring programs (PDMPs). The American Dental Education Association and the US Substance Abuse and Mental Health Services Administration cosponsored the Dental Schools Addiction Summit on the Opioid Epidemic in 2017 to discuss opioid epidemic trends and share strategies for preventing prescription drug abuse and addiction.

This issue of *Dental Clinics of North America* provides a resource for everyone involved in the care of dental patients. The 10 articles in the issue provide the reader with the background and resources needed to be a competent clinician in dealing with patients in pain while contributing to the end of the epidemic. The article by Dhadwal and colleagues sets the stage by providing a historical overview of dentistry's role in assessing and managing the complex patient at risk for substance abuse and "best practices." The article by Schatman and colleagues focuses on the patient interview and developing strategies to identify substance abuse disorders. Keith and Hernández-Nuño de la Rosa provide information on special screening resources available to the clinician, including PDMPs. Khawaja and Scrivani focus on managing acute dental pain, including options for pain management using drugs other than opioids. Fortino and colleagues identify medical and psychiatric conditions associated with increased risk of abuse and misuse. Viswanath and colleagues in their article deal with perhaps the most complex patient: the high-risk dental patient with active substance abuse disorder. Acknowledging that there are opportunities for motivational intervention, Schatman and Shapiro identify strategies for the successful management of the complex, nonadherent dental patient. Dentists are not alone in coping with complex patients, and Kulich and Keith provide strategies for appropriate interactions between dentists and other health care providers. The article by Magee addresses special high-risk populations in dentistry, including adolescents, the elderly, and women of childbearing age. The article by Keith and colleagues provides critical information on ways in which dentists can effectively manage legal liability risks and the responsible prescription of controlled substances for patients in need.

The audience for this issue is not just practicing dentists. Consider the amount of time that many dental patients spend with a dental hygienist and, in some states, with a dental therapist. Sharing the concepts contained within this issue with other professionals in the dental office will help the entire dental team to be sensitive to the complexities of patients in dental pain, and the roles that they can play in identifying those patients who are seeking prescription drugs that they may misuse or abuse.

Much of this issue focuses on enhancing interviewing, screening, and motivational skills for dentists in identifying and counseling patients who need or are seeking prescription medications. These skills don't always come naturally to dentists, whose education and training have made them experts at dental diagnosis and treatment planning but not always as strong at communicating with patients and other health care providers. During my tenure as the CEO of the American Dental Education Association, I also served concurrently as President of the Interprofessional Education Collaborative. Also known as IPEC, this coalition of 20 associations represents schools of the health professions. Our initial priority was to develop competencies for interprofessional education and collaborative care. Early in our meetings, it became clear that one of the major barriers to collaboration was the fact that each profession has its own vocabulary, with each one using words and phrases common to their individual profession but not always easily understood by providers in other professions. One of the key elements of this issue of Dental Clinics of North America is the way in which health care professionals interact with each other to enhance the care of patients they share. Given that the authors of this issue include dentists, oral and maxillofacial surgeons, physicians, psychiatrists, behavioral scientists, anesthesiologists, pain experts, and researchers, this should not be a surprise. This will have a significant impact on the way we approach not only patients in pain but also all patients that we care for in collaboration in the future.

Richard W. Valachovic, DMD, MPH
New York University College of Dentistry
345 East 24th Street
New York, NY 10010, USA

*E-mail address:*
valachovicrw@gmail.com

## REFERENCES

1. Suda KJ, Durkin MJ, Calip GS, et al. Comparison of opioid prescribing by dentists in the United States and England. JAMA Netw Open 2019;2(5):e194303. https://doi.org/10.1001/jamanetworkopen.2019.4303.
2. National Institute of Drug Abuse. Opioid overdose crisis. 2019. Available at: https://www.drugabuse.gov/drugs-abuse/opioids/opioid-overdose-crisis. Accessed January 4, 2020.
3. American Dental Association. Opioid prescribing by dentists. 2016. Available at: https://www.ada.org/~/media/ADA/Advocacy/Files/Opioids%202018_ADA%20HPI_Opioids%20Perscribing%20by%20Dentists.pdf?la=en. Accessed January 4, 2020.
4. Keith DA, Kulich RJ, Bharel M, et al. Massachusetts dental schools respond to the prescription opioid crisis: a statewide collaboration. J Dent Educ 2017;81:1388–94.
5. Dye BA, Xianfen L, Beltran-Aguilar ED. Selected oral health indicators in the United States 2005-2008. NCHS data brief no. 96. Hyattsville (MD): National Center for Health Statistics, Centers for Disease Control and Prevention; 2012.
6. Eke P, Thornton-Evans G, Wei L, et al. Periodontitis in US adults: National Health and Nutrition Examination Survey 2009-2014. J Am Dent Assoc 2018;149:576–86.
7. American Dental Association. 2005-06 Survey of dental services rendered. Chicago (IL): 2007.

# Dentistry's Role in Assessing and Managing Controlled Substance Risk

## Historical Overview, Current Barriers, and Working Toward Best Practices

Shuchi Dhadwal, DMD[a],*, Ronald J. Kulich, PhD[a,b],
Priyanka Monga, DDS[a], Michael E. Schatman, PhD[a,c]

### KEYWORDS

- Controlled substances • Opioids • Barriers to care • Collaborative treatment
- Opioid use disorder

### KEY POINTS

- Dentistry is in a unique position among the health care professions to assess and manage the patient with controlled substance risk.
- The concern over opioid risk is not new, and historically dentists have had to balance the critical need for adequate pain care with the importance of recognizing the consequences of using controlled substances for their patients.
- Barriers for providing adequate patient assessment and management may be greater in dentistry than other health care fields, although these barriers can be recognized and overcome.
- Collaboration with cotreating providers will improve patient outcomes and reduce patient risk.

According to the Centers for Disease Control and Prevention, in 2017, 17.4% of the US population received 1 or more opioid prescriptions, with the average patient receiving 3.4 prescriptions.[1] This figure decreased dramatically in 2018. Based on a 2019 IQVIA report,[2] opioid prescribing decreased by 17.1% from 2017 to 2018, with a decrease of 43% since the peak in 2011. Although this decrease is encouraging, considerable work is still left to be done. Given the outcries by patients and the health care

[a] Department of Diagnostic Sciences, Tufts University School of Dental Medicine, 1 Kneeland Street, Boston, MA 02111, USA; [b] Department of Anesthesia, Critical Care and Pain Medicine, Harvard Medical School, Massachusetts General Hospital, Boston, MA, USA; [c] Department of Public Health and Community Medicine, Tufts University School of Medicine, Boston, MA, USA
* Corresponding author.
*E-mail address:* shuchi.dhadwal@tufts.edu

Dent Clin N Am 64 (2020) 491–501
https://doi.org/10.1016/j.cden.2020.02.002
0011-8532/20/© 2020 Elsevier Inc. All rights reserved.

professionals who care for them,[3–5] a better balance should be achieved between the need to provide effective and safe analgesia and the societal obligation to avoid a turn to previous prescribing habits and the consequences of such.

Despite the desire to attribute the prescription opioid crisis to a single cause, there are, in fact, numerous causes of the prescription opioid epidemic. The recent report from the President's Commission on Combating Drug Addiction and the Opioid Crisis noted that "the root causes of the modern opioid crisis are complex and traceable to at least 30 or more factors."[6] Fortunately, the prescription opioid crisis has declined, although it has been replaced by a crisis of far more deadly illicit opioids. Controversies regarding opioids in pain management seem to have become more salient in regard to chronic pain rather than acute pain.[7,8] Irrespective, extreme caution in opioid prescribing still needs to be exercised, even in the field of dentistry in which acute pain management remains the primary focus.

For acute dental pain, the relative effectiveness of nonsteroidal anti-inflammatory drugs have received insufficient attention, because there was level of comfort with prescribing opioids. Even vulnerable populations such as adolescents have been routinely and repeatedly prescribed opioids for conditions such as migraine headache and other pain-related disorders for which there is little evidence of treatment efficacy, and often contraindication.[9] All of these efforts, at least in part, were thought to contribute to what had been termed a prescription opioid epidemic in the United States. Significant social, economic, individual, and family impacts have been widely reported and discussed, although newer shifts in prescribing practices and other factors are now seen as relieving the problem.[10]

Within the past several years, the opioid prescribing rates for all health care specialists have decreased, particularly in dentistry. In 2017, prescription opioids continued to contribute to the epidemic in the United States, with data from the Centers for Disease Control and Prevention suggesting that they were involved in more than 35% of all opioid overdose deaths.[11] It should be noted that the methods that Centers for Disease Control and Prevention used to determine this number were likely flawed, resulting in an overstatement of the percentage of total opioid deaths accurately attributable to prescription opioid overdoses.[12] Irrespective, improved opioid risk mitigation, including frequent urine drug screening, use of prescription drug monitoring programs (PDMPs), and easier access to naloxone is likely to have had a positive impact on prescription opioid misuse associated morbidity and mortality.[4] Nonetheless, individuals with severe opioid use disorders risk have shifted to street-acquired drugs, owing to the decreased availability of prescription opioids that can be used for abuse in conjunction with the considerably lower relative costs of heroin and illicit fentanyl and its analogues.[13] Some investigators believe that recent deaths can be attributed to polypharmacy, that is, a mix of legal substances, in conjunction with diverted controlled substances and/or illicit substances, rather than solely medications from the prescribing physician or dentist.[14]

## OPIOIDS AND DENTISTRY

Although general dentistry was somewhat less impacted by the early direct marketing efforts, the right to pain relief efforts did provide tacit permission to ignore opioid prescribing risks. Dentists rarely prescribed long-acting agents, and seldom prescribed short-acting agents for long periods of time. There are examples of high numbers of short-acting opioids after surgical procedures such as third molar extractions. At 1 point, dentistry was second after primary care physicians in prescribing overall quantities of short-acting opioids.[15]

Potentially complicating the problem, some investigators have suggested that there have also been excessive surgical treatments, particularly in young adults, resulting in their needless exposure to opioids.[16] In a retrospective cohort study, Schroeder and colleagues[16] found that a substantial number of adolescents are exposed to opioid prescriptions after third molar extractions. They postulated that opioid-naïve young patients were at a higher risk of opioid use/misuse with this sort of exposure. Historically, these concerns have been more common in other procedure-based health care disciplines, with data demonstrating that 1 in 16 surgical patients becomes a long-term user after being prescribed opioids for a surgical procedure.[17] In an attempt to mitigate this problem, national efforts have been undertaken to decrease the number of controlled substances prescribed to patients upon discharge from the hospital, as postsurgical opioid use has been established as a predictor of increased readmission rates and higher risk of substance abuse.[18]

## SUBSTANCE USE DISORDERS

In contrast with other substance use disorders, opioid use disorder has received greater attention over the past several years. Despite this attention, alcohol abuse and other types of substance abuse are more commonly seen in health care settings,[19] including general dental practice. Furthermore, patients with polysubstance use issues are at greater risk. Hence, all types of substance use and abuse deserve close attention by dentists who see these patients in their practice on a daily basis.

The Substance Abuse and Mental Health Services Administration states that "substance use disorders occur when the recurrent use of alcohol and/or drugs causes clinically significant impairment, including health problems, disability, and failure to meet major responsibilities at work, school, or home."[20] Although more detailed diagnostic criteria are reviewed in later chapters and available elsewhere (eg, the *Diagnostic and Statistical Manual of Mental Disorders,* 5th editions), the broad-based description from the Substance Abuse and Mental Health Services Administration best fits the appropriate lay definition of substance abuse. Substance use disorders are classified as a brain disease, with a focus on minimizing the common stigma associated with the illness. As with any chronic disease, multiple treatment trials may be necessary, but recovery is often possible with proper treatment, regardless of the severity of the illness.

When any substance use disorder is present, the patient's status is also often complicated by the coexistence of mental health disorders. Substance use disorder is rarely a stand-alone illness, necessitating a broader scope of patient assessment.[21] In this series, we strongly encourage the dentist to devote attention to the mental health comorbidities often present in patients with high substance use risk. Data from the Substance Abuse and Mental Health Services Administration underscore this overlap (**Fig. 1**).

Common substance use disorders seen within dental practice include alcohol, nicotine, and more recently cannabis use disorders, and each is associated with an array of dental and medical consequences. Among adults age 18 and older in 2018, 14.4 million adults or 5.8% of the age group suffer from an alcohol use disorder, with fewer than 8% receiving treatment.[22] Alcohol abuse remains the third leading preventable cause of death in the United States, the first being tobacco, the second being poor diet and physical inactivity.[23] Tobacco abuse, a disorder commonly addressed in dentistry, predicts a higher likelihood of opioid misuse in the context of treating chronic pain.[24] Similarly, the mere presence of cannabis in a patient's urine predicts a higher likelihood of subsequent aberrant urine toxicology screening when chronic

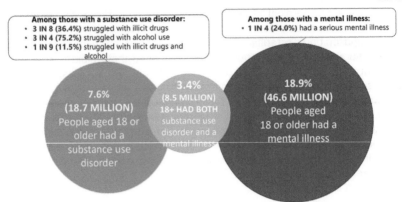

**Fig. 1.** Mental and substance use disorders in America. (*From* Substance Abuse and Mental Health Services Administration. The 2017-18 national survey on drug use and health. Available at: https://www.samhsa.gov/data/sites/default/files/nsduh-ppt-09-2018.pdf. Accessed on January 26, 2020.)

opioids are being prescribed.[25] Given the interrelationship of these comorbid risk factors, predicting patient behavior associated with substance abuse is challenging. Nonetheless, cost-effective screening in the dental office can provide the dentist with important information, resulting in improved patient management, and the patient may be offered more efficient referral and access to effective treatment.

## HISTORICAL ANTECEDENTS TO MANAGING PAIN AND ADDRESSING SUBSTANCE USE RISK

Dentistry now plays an important role in the management of the patient's overall health, with national organizations such as the American Dental Association and the American Dental Education Association increasingly highlighting the need for responsible assessment of substance use risk and better management of these complex patients.[26] Most important, this effort must be balanced with adequate pain care for the patient. Although some may believe that concern over the balance between substance use risk and effective pain management is new, they have been voiced in dentistry for more than a century.

Since its inception as a health care specialty, dentistry has played a crucial role in acute pain management and analgesia. The first successful public demonstration of ether for surgical purposes was provided by the dentist William Thomas Morton at Massachusetts General Hospital on October 16, 1846. Horace Wells and other dentists also were using similar agents to care for their patients years before. As ether moved from a recreational frolic drug toward common medical use, surgeries dramatically increased in number across the United States and Europe. Concurrent with the famous anesthesia demonstration, opioids were coming into widespread use throughout the nineteenth century to better manage pain for a range of conditions, including acute dental pain. Not unlike today's controversies, national debates ensued regarding the role of opioids and the prescription of other potentially risky substances by physicians and dentists, and discussions of industry influence and physician bias were as common then as they are today.[27] In 1891, Oliver Wendell Holmes Sr., the famed physician and anatomist from Harvard, was widely quoted in newspapers across the country when he stated "if a ship-load of miscellaneous drugs, with certain very important exceptions, drugs, many of which were then often given needlessly and in excess, as then used could be sunk to the bottom of the sea, it would be all the better for mankind and all the worse for the fishes."[27] Because of lack of regulations of drugs such as opioids and cocaine, there was widespread opioid prescribing for multiple conditions. To decrease the sudden increase of drug dependence, the Harrison Narcotic Control Act was passed in 1914. Nonetheless, the concerns did not abate.

Historically, the twentieth century witnessed better control of acute pain with a range of effective strategies for analgesia and anesthesia. Effective nonopioid analgesics were introduced, especially agents such as acetaminophen and nonsteroidal anti-inflammatory drugs (see Shehryar Nasir Khawaja and Steven John Scrivani's article, "Managing Acute Dental Pain: Principles for Rational Prescribing and Alternatives to Opioid Therapy," in this issue).

## PROVIDING ADEQUATE PAIN MANAGEMENT AND CONCURRENT ASSESSMENT OF RISK

Safe and effective pain management is critical in dentistry, particularly in acute pain management. Echoing guidance from all professional organizations, the Dental Education Core Competencies for the Prevention and Management of Prescription Drug Misuse note that "dentists deal predominantly with acute pain, using standard evaluations and evidence-based treatment protocols that are highly effective for acute pain."[28] This is now commonly termed "rational prescribing." Rational prescribing does not mean "not prescribing."[29] In addition to selecting safer and more effective nonopioid agents when appropriate, interventional and nonpharmacologic strategies also can play a role. Assessing risk, knowing the patient, and setting realistic patient expectation can also help to guide decision making.

Although other articles in this special issue provide more detailed guidance with specific detailed case vignettes, the case of a 19-year-old woman illustrates a common scenario of low to moderate controlled substance risk. She presented for an urgent dental visit and was a longstanding patient in the practice with the patient and her family being well-known to the dentist and staff. Her previous office visit had been approximately 1 year prior, with irregular follow-up, partially owing to a recent job loss and insurance change. The assistant fit her in for an evaluation of her new complaint of dental pain before the weekend. An initial thorough examination and assessment revealed a diagnosis of irreversible pulpitis, with a treatment recommendation for a pulpectomy on #21. Because she had not been seen for more than a year, diligent reassessment by the dental hygienist revealed that the patient was taking hydrocodone and diazepam prescribed by her primary care physician, with the dosing being unclear. The patient stated that "my medications are mostly the same, except for some changes in my headache and neck pain medications. I had been using a little bit of Vicodin for my neck, but it hasn't helped with this new dental problem. I use a little bit of diazepam as it gets me through the night." She further revealed that she occasionally used "a few Fioricet, a couple per month for my migraines. I'm not on any other medications." In the conversation with the dentist, her social history revealed that she had a strong social support system, a stable relationship, and planned marriage soon.

As with most patients, this dentist had a good rapport with the patient who was well-known to the practice. A narrow approach could have been pursued, finalizing plans for the dental procedure, and the patient could have been discharged with the standard follow-up. Strong analgesics would unlikely have been needed, and the patient's care could have been managed with a short-term nonsteroidal anti-inflammatory drug. Despite this common care scenario, the case presented the dentist with an opportunity to more thoroughly address opioid risk. As discussed in greater detail in articles elsewhere in this issue, this patient presented with a number of substance use risk factors that required further assessment. Although her opioids were apparently low dose, she admitted to using an opioid left over from another prescription for a dental problem, a condition for which the medication was not prescribed. Additionally, she was concurrently using 3 controlled substances (an opioid, a benzodiazepine, and a barbiturate), a factor that can increase risk. Although the dentist may not have been mandated to check the PDMP because a prescription for opioids was not as yet planned, it was a reasonable option to consider a PDMP check before initiating the dental procedure. In this case, the check revealed that she had had 1 prescription from her primary care physician filled 11 months prior for hydrocodone/acetaminophen 325/5 mg, #10 with no refills, with no other opioids listed. She was prescribed and filled diazepam 2 mg #45/mo on an ongoing basis from primary care, and her most recent Fioricet prescription for 30 tablets had been refilled 6 months prior. These PDMP results were consistent with her self-report. As part of the reassessment, the hygienist also administered a brief self-report substance use screener, on which the patient denied abuse of other substances other than for smoking less than 1 pack of cigarettes per day. This young woman's case is relatively common to most dental practices. Further discussion revealed risk factors that often go unnoticed. She had polypharmacy issues and was using opioids for a problem for which they were not prescribed, that is, her recent dental pain. Her risks were further heightened in that she may have been experiencing stressors associated with a recent job loss. Even at low dosages, she remained on a medication regimen that posed additional risks for women of childbearing age, should she have become pregnant. It also was noted that she was smoking, representing a risk factor that is predictive of other substance use disorders, including an opioid use disorder. The patient's positive relationship with the dentist provided a unique opportunity for further assessment and management. Even if the dentist merely made note of these risk factors and supportively addressed these concerns, there is an opportunity to exert a substantive impact on the patient's overall health care and well-being. This discussion typically builds on the positive relationship between the patient and clinician. Despite their sensitivity, such personal discussions also predict better general adherence with other dental treatment recommendations, and thus overall treatment outcomes may be improved. This factor is discussed in an article in this issue on the importance of actual discussion as opposed to mere questioning in communicating with patients.

Throughout this issue, we discuss assessment protocols that can guide the dentist in evaluating patients who may have a low to a high risk of substance misuse. Although an increasing number of standardized risk screeners are available for physicians, we have elected to focus on practical strategies that are more likely to fit general dental practice (**Fig. 2**). It is not expected that the dentist would cover every risk factor for all patients. The very complex, high-risk patient may be well-served with the most thorough assessment, that is, covering all of the assessment components addressed in **Fig. 2**. Consultation and referral with an addiction medicine specialist should be considered an option in cases in which substantial risk is present. Finally, the role of the dental hygienist cannot be discounted. Indeed, it is not uncommon for the hygienist to have the closest relationship with the patient, and they can effectively use the brief risk screeners outlined in additional articles in this issue.

| Comprehensive risk assessment: | Data from other sources: |
|---|---|
| [Steps to gather information and begin to formulate an understanding of the patient's medical, psychosocial, and substance use risk] | [Additional sources of information that may be critical to an accurate risk assessment] |
| ✓ Provide rationale for questions/risk assessment<br>✓ Assess pain<br>✓ Assess current substance use, including legal and illicit substances<br>✓ *Assess medical and psychosocial risk factors*<br>✓ Assess dental risk factors<br>✓ *Analyze relevant physical exam and/or mental health findings* | ✓ *Check PMP and interpret findings*<br>✓ Complete screening questionnaires (NIDA quick-screen)<br>✓ *Communicate with other treating clinicians*<br>✓ *Communicate with patient and family members/caregivers* |

| Disposition & follow-up care: | Ongoing collaboration & (re)assessment |
|---|---|
| [Steps for documentation, patient education/informed consent, and appropriate follow-up care, including referrals] | [Steps that ensure communication and coordination between providers; consideration of special needs and on-going assessment of at-risk patients] |
| ✓ Determine/document level of risk prior to prescribing<br>✓ Individualized treatment recommendations<br>✓ Determine likelihood of adherence/follow-up<br>✓ *Make appropriate referrals: MH, SA, pain care*<br>✓ Instruct patient re: safe Rx disposal<br>✓ *Assess need for continued monitoring and/or higher level of care*<br>✓ *Document in chart, including PMP assessment, communications, and referrals* | ✓ *Communicate and collaborate with other care providers*<br>✓ Perform periodic reassessment of pain, SUD risk, and mental health comorbidities<br>✓ Attend to special at-risk populations: The patient in SUD recovery, the patient requiring naloxone, adolescents, pregnancy, etc. |

**Fig. 2.** Controlled substance risk mitigation (CSRM) checklist. NIDA, National Institute on Drug Abuse; PMP, prescription monitoring program; Rx, prescription; SUD, substance use disorder.

## BARRIERS TO RISK ASSESSMENT AND SCREENING IN DENTISTRY

Dentists are in a unique position to address substance use risk, because they often see their patients more frequently than do their primary care providers and may have more direct, face-to-face contact time. Owing to the structure of the current health care system in the United States, patients may change physicians with considerable frequency, whereas their relationships with their dentists and dental hygienists often remain stable. Despite this unique position, serious barriers exist with respect to conducting an adequate substance use risk assessment in dentistry.

Until recently, there has been limited research on the topic of substance use risk screening in dentistry. The results of a cross-sectional survey study conducted by the CDC National Center for Injury Prevention and Control[1] revealed that very few dentists regularly screen for prescription drug abuse or request prior medical records. They also reported that there are significant gaps that exist in dental training in the assessment of prescription opioid misuse and diversion. Investigators in dentistry are only recently exploring these gaps in practice, with most studies occurring within the past 5 years. Similarly, the dental hygiene literature offers little direction with respect to current or proposed practice guidelines for substance use risk assessment. Current screenings in general dental practices typically involve the completion a self-report standard medical history form, which may include 1 or 2 items on substance use. This abbreviated approach typically fails to cover the full range of risk factors and often does not bring the patient into any conversation with the clinician regarding risk.

Exposure to training in substance risk assessment and management can be critically important, even though attitudes may be slow to change. Parish and colleagues[30] determined that dentists who had prior experience and knowledge regarding substance misuse were more likely to inquire about patients' histories of substance use/misuse and more receptive to using screening tools in their clinical practices. Past dental education efforts on this topic have been chiefly lecture based, although there are newer programs that include an interprofessional mix of students from dentistry, pharmacy, and medicine with the use of simulated cases. Ronald J. Kulich and colleagues' article, "Interprofessional Collaboration in the Assessment and Management of Substance Use Risk," in this issue reviews an interprofessional program that provides students with training in controlled substance risk mitigation and naloxone education, although supporting research on its effectiveness is still needed.

Dental continuing education training may also be a barrier. Currently, most required dentistry continuing education training is centered on physician-based educational programs, whereby dentists are commonly exposed to clinical scenarios that involve the assessment and monitoring of patients on chronic opioid therapy or the use of urine toxicology evaluations. This type of focus may be helpful for the small number of oral and maxillofacial surgeons and orofacial pain dentists who treat chronic pain and use long-acting opioids, yet offers little practical advice for general dental practice.

Attitudes and related stigma about substance use also persist. Parish and colleagues[30] concluded that approximately two-thirds of dentists did not believe that screening for substance use was compatible with their professional roles. Even clinicians with expertise in substance use disorder assessment or pain medicine do not consistently appreciate the potential role of dentistry in substance abuse risk mitigation, a barrier discussed in the article on interprofessional care in this issue. As medicine has evolved into multiple subspecialties, a common retort is heard, "I didn't sign up to be a psychiatrist," a critical comment also occasionally heard from young dentists-in-training who still view their role as executing procedures. Similarly, even subspecialty practices in orofacial pain, an area of study in which there is a high risk for substance use disorder and mental health comorbidities among their patients, still rarely follow Academy of Orofacial Pain guidance with respect to the use standardized behavioral screening and outcome measures. In part, these attitudes and behaviors are likely influenced by concerns over time burden, lack of comfort with a sensitive subject matter, or the stigma associated with individuals suffering from substance use disorders. The article in this issue on motivational interviewing describes specific techniques that can help to decrease clinician anxiety with respect to addressing sensitive subject matter. Eventually, the shift toward larger interprofessional practice may help to improve clinician comfort and decrease biases potentially evident in the assessment and management of these patients.

Electronic dental records are another substantial handicap, and the article on interprofessional care by Ronald J. Kulich and colleagues' article, "Interprofessional Collaboration in the Assessment and Management of Substance Use Risk," in this issue outlines this barrier in greater detail. Most dental record systems cannot easily accommodate standardized screening assessments, and there are few user-friendly templates for addressing the medical and psychiatric comorbidities commonly seen among patients with substance use disorders. Additionally, medical record access presents another major barrier. Physicians and substance use disorder specialists can readily view each other's notes, which can facilitate efficient communication. In contrast, dental records are typically unavailable to physicians and medical records cannot be easily accessed by dentists. Communication is universally critical for effective evaluation and management of the complex patient, and health care records can provide an important resource for facilitating that communication.

Finally, there are concerns regarding Health Insurance Portability and Accountability Act of 1996 (HIPAA) barriers pertaining to record exchange or communication across treatment providers. These barriers are often overstated, because there are few HIPAA restrictions for cross-communicating with cotreating providers. Nonetheless, transparency is the best rule, requiring entering into discussions with patients regarding the importance of conferring with other providers.

## STRUCTURED GUIDANCE FOR ASSISTING THE PRACTICING DENTIST

The goals of assessing risk within dentistry are inherently different and more circumscribed than are those in primary care, pain medicine, and other types of medical practices in which the clinician provides direct substance use disorder care. Although the practicing dentist may greatly benefit by have an increased knowledge regarding current treatment protocols for substance use assessment and care, few will prescribe medication-assisted treatment for opioid abuse, interpreting risk through analysis of urine toxicology, or providing other therapies for substance use disorders. Where possible, screening questionnaires should have an adequate empirical basis with normative and predictive validity data collected from dental settings. Research remains limited in this area, and there remains an urge to adopt assessment approaches intended for physicians. For example, a group of medical deans and several state officials from Massachusetts suggested that the local dental schools adopt controlled substance risk curriculum guidelines developed for use in the region's medical schools. After an initial review of the documents, the dental task force, proposed more relevant dentist-friendly training guidelines, "Governor's Dental Education Working Group on Prescription Drug Misuse." This group produced the Dental Education Core Competencies for the Prevention and Management of Prescription Drug Misuse, a document that help to guide the application of this initial series of papers.[31]

## SERIES SUMMARY AND FUTURE DIRECTIONS

Building on the initial work noted in this article, we also drew content from the June 8, 2019, Interprofessional Controlled Substance Risk Mitigation Initiative Symposium. This interactive forum held at Tufts University School of Dental Medicine brought together dentists, oral surgeons, physicians, dental hygienists, students, and other content experts from medical, nursing, and psychiatric/psychological fields. With training modules still in development and testing, this series of articles mirrors much of the content of this special issue.

The articles in this issue cover the identification of psychiatric and medical risk factors, strategies for motivational interviewing with complex dental patients, using standardized screeners and state PDMPs, pharmacotherapeutic management of acute dental pain, and strategies for management and referral of low-, medium- and high-risk patients. Because patient populations such as adolescents may be at greater risk, the need for special attention to those groups is also addressed. Finally, when dealing with complex patients, there is always a need to address areas of liability risk, scope of practice, and documentation. Despite the constant regulatory changes that occur, David A. Keith and colleagues' article, "Opioid Prescribing in Dental Practice: Managing Liability Risks," in this issue provides practice advice for reducing risk for the patient, as well as medicolegal and regulatory risks for the provider.

Although dentists may be writing fewer opioid prescriptions and decreasing the number of doses that are prescribed, the assessment and management of substance use risk must also become a mainstay of care. There remain a broad range of barriers impacting adequate assessment and management of controlled substance risk. It is hoped that this issue results in these barriers gradually becoming adequately managed.

## DISCLOSURE

Partial support was received for the preparation of this article through a grant from "The Coverys Community Healthcare Foundation".

## REFERENCES

1. CDC National Center for Injury Prevention and Control. Annual surveillance report of drug-related risks and outcomes, United States, 2018. Available at: https://www.cdc.gov/drugoverdose/pdf/pubs/2018-cdc-drug-surveillance-report.pdf. Accessed January 19, 2020.

2. IQVIA Institute. Medicine use and spending in the U.S.: a review of 2018 and outlook to 2023. 2019. Available at: https://www.iqvia.com/insights/the-iqvia-institute/reports/medicine-use-and-spending-in-the-us-a-review-of-2018-and-outlook-to-2023. Accessed January 28, 2020.

3. Kertesz SG, Gordon AJ. A crisis of opioids and the limits of prescription control: United States. Addiction 2019;114(1):169–80.

4. Schatman ME, Vasciannie A, Kulich RJ. Opioid moderatism and the imperative of rapprochement in pain medicine. J Pain Res 2019;12:849–57.

5. Brennan MJ, Gudin JA. The prescription opioid conundrum: 21st century solutions to a millennia-long problem. Postgrad Med 2019;1–11. https://doi.org/10.1080/00325481.2019.1677383.

6. Madras BK. The president's commission on combating drug addiction and the opioid crisis: origins and recommendations. Clin Pharmacol Ther 2018;103(6):943–5.

7. Volkow N, Benveniste H, McLellan AT. Use and misuse of opioids in chronic pain. Annu Rev Med 2018;69:451–65.

8. Tucker HR, Scaff K, McCloud T, et al. Harms and benefits of opioids for management of non-surgical acute and chronic low back pain: a systematic review. Br J Sports Med 2019. https://doi.org/10.1136/bjsports-2018-099805 [pii:bjsports-2018-099805].

9. Edlund MJ, Martin BC, Russo JE, et al. The role of opioid prescription in incident opioid abuse and dependence among individuals with chronic noncancer pain: the role of opioid prescription. Clin J Pain 2014;30(7):557–64.

10. Florence CS, Zhou C, Luo F, et al. The Economic burden of prescription opioid overdose, abuse, and dependence in the United States, 2013. Med Care 2016;54(10):901–6.

11. United States Centers for Disease Control and Prevention. Overdose death maps: overdose deaths involving prescription opioids. Available at: https://www.cdc.gov/drugoverdose/data/prescribing/overdose-death-maps.html. Accessed January 29, 2020.

12. Schatman ME, Ziegler SJ. Pain management, prescription opioid mortality, and the CDC: is the devil in the data? J Pain Res 2017;10:2489–95.

13. Surratt HL, Kurtz SP, Buttram M, et al. Heroin use onset among nonmedical prescription opioid users in the club scene. Drug Alcohol Depend 2017;179:131–8.

14. Eisenberg MD, Saloner B, Krawczyk N, et al. Use of opioid overdose deaths reported in one state's criminal justice, hospital, and prescription databases to identify risk of opioid fatalities. JAMA Intern Med 2019;179(7):980–2.

15. Volkow ND, McLellan TA, Cotto JH, et al. Characteristics of opioid prescriptions in 2009. JAMA 2011;305(13):1299–301.
16. Schroeder AR, Dehghan M, Newman TB, et al. Association of opioid prescriptions from dental clinicians for US adolescents and young adults with subsequent opioid use and abuse. JAMA Intern Med 2019;179(2):145–52.
17. Overton HN, Hanna MN, Bruhn WE, et al. Opioid-prescribing guidelines for common surgical procedures: an expert panel consensus. J Am Coll Surg 2018; 227(4):411–8.
18. Hill MV, Stucke RS, McMahon ML, et al. An Educational intervention decreases opioid prescribing after general surgical operations. Ann Surg 2018;267(3):468–72.
19. Cherpitel CJ, Ye Y. Drug use and problem drinking associated with primary care and emergency room utilization in the US general population: data from the 2005 national alcohol survey. Drug Alcohol Depend 2008;97:226–30.
20. Lipari RNVHS. Trends in Substance Use Disorders Among Adults Aged 18 or Older. The CBHSQ Report. Rockville (MD): Substance Abuse and Mental Health Services Administration (US); 2013-. Available at: https://www.ncbi.nlm.nih.gov/books/NBK447253/2017. Accessed January 29, 2020.
21. Compton WM, Thomas YF, Stinson FS, et al. Prevalence, correlates, disability, and comorbidity of DSM-IV drug abuse and dependence in the United States: results from the national epidemiologic survey on alcohol and related conditions. Arch Gen Psychiatry 2007;64(5):566–76.
22. United States Substance Abuse and Mental Health Services Administration. Key substance use and mental health indicators in the United States: results from the 2018 National Survey on Drug Use and Health, August, 2019. Available at: https://www.samhsa.gov/data/sites/default/files/cbhsq-reports/NSDUHNationalFindingsReport2018/NSDUHNationalFindingsReport2018.pdf. Accessed January 29, 2020.
23. National Institute on Alcohol Abuse and Alcoholism. Alcohol Facts and Statistics. 2019. Available at: https://www.niaaa.nih.gov/publications/brochures-and-fact-sheets/alcohol-facts-and-statistics. Accessed January 29, 2020.
24. Coyle DT, Pratt CY, Ocran-Appiah J, et al. Opioid analgesic dose and the risk of misuse, overdose, and death: a narrative review. Pharmacoepidemiol Drug Saf 2018;27(5):464–72.
25. DiBenedetto DJ, Weed VF, Wawrzyniak KM, et al. The association between cannabis use and aberrant behaviors during chronic opioid therapy for chronic pain. Pain Med 2018;19(10):1997–2008.
26. American Dental Association. Substance use disorders. Available at: https://www.ada.org/en/advocacy/current-policies/substance-use-disorders. Accessed January 29, 2020.
27. Kulich R, Loeser JD. The business of pain medicine: the present mirrors antiquity. Pain Med 2011;12(7):1063–75.
28. Antman KH, Berman HA, Flotte TR, et al. Developing core competencies for the prevention and management of prescription drug misuse: a medical education collaboration in Massachusetts. Acad Med 2016;91(10):1348–51.
29. Fischer MA, Avorn J. Step therapy-clinical algorithms, legislation, and optimal prescribing. JAMA 2017;317(8):801–2.
30. Parish CL, Pereyra MR, Pollack HA, et al. Screening for substance misuse in the dental care setting: findings from a nationally representative survey of dentists. Addiction 2015;110(9):1516–23.
31. Keith DA, Kulich RJ, Bharel M, et al. Massachusetts dental schools respond to the prescription opioid crisis: a statewide collaboration. J Dent Educ 2017;81(12):1388–94.

# Patient Interviewing Strategies to Recognize Substance Use, Misuse, and Abuse in the Dental Setting

Michael E. Schatman, PhD[a,b],*, Ellen Patterson, MD[c],
Hannah Shapiro[d]

## KEYWORDS

- Clinical interviewing • Substance use risk • Substance use screening

## KEY POINTS

- Substance use risk screening is an important element of the comprehensive dental assessment and relevant to safety of anesthesia, medication interactions, pain management, and the assessment of oral health risk factors.
- Validated screening tools may be administered verbally, as a written checklist, or online by various members of the dental team; they can serve as an entry point for gathering detailed information, when appropriate.
- Dental practitioners can apply widely accepted interviewing approaches that foster mutual trust, enhance communication, encourage patient engagement, and improve patient satisfaction with the clinical encounter.
- A dental team–based approach to risk assessment can be used to overcome challenges, such as lack of time.

## INTERVIEWING FOR SCREENING AND RISK ASSESSMENT

Oral health clinicians have long been trained to apply data from patient interviews to risk assessments that are relevant to oral health. For example, early empirical literature determined that clinical interviews that included a dietary history were more effective for assessing caries risk and enabled the clinician to give specific dietary advice in quantitative terms.[1] Because patients expect oral health providers to ask questions

[a] Department of Diagnostic Sciences, Tufts University School of Dental Medicine, 1 Kneeland Street, Boston, MA 02111, USA; [b] Department of Public Health & Community Medicine, Tufts University School of Medicine, Boston, MA, USA; [c] Department of Comprehensive Care, Tufts University School of Dental Medicine, 1 Kneeland Street, Boston, MA 02111, USA; [d] Department of Biopsychology, Tufts University, Robinson Hall, 200 College Avenue, Medford, MA 02155, USA
* Corresponding author.
E-mail address: Michael.Schatman@tufts.edu

Dent Clin N Am 64 (2020) 503–512
https://doi.org/10.1016/j.cden.2020.02.001
0011-8532/20/© 2020 Elsevier Inc. All rights reserved.

regarding oral hygiene and dietary habits, they are unlikely to react negatively to these interview topics, as the relevance to their oral health is clear. However, patients may be initially reluctant to answer similarly probing questions regarding alcohol and other substance use habits, because these topics are potentially awkward, stigmatizing, and may seem unrelated to oral health. This is especially true if the interviewer does not make explicit to the patient the relevant clinical connections between substance use and health risks relevant to dental practice.

Some oral health providers incorporate self-report questionnaires or brief interview-based screeners to gather patient information regarding current and past substance use (a topic that is further addressed in the David A. Keith and María F. Hernández-Nuño de la Rosa's article, "Special Screening Resources: Strategies to Identify Substance Use Disorders, Including Opioid Misuse and Abuse", elsewhere in this issue). Brief validated substance use screeners may be easily integrated within the health history–taking process in dental settings and can provide valuable information in a relatively short time. The dentist (or another member of the dental team) may administer these screeners while collecting or updating other health history data. Screeners are most effective when they are administered as an aspect of the routine practice flow to all adult patients, as clinicians are typically poor predictors of patients at greater risk of substance use disorders based solely on demographic information. Routine screening also helps to dispel stigma, especially if the clinician emphasizes the safety considerations of alcohol, prescription drugs, and other substance use for dental anesthesia, drug interactions, and potential impact on oral health risks. **Table 1** lists several commonly used and evidence-based screening tools, with links to their online versions for easy reference.

The US Preventive Services Task Force currently recommends screening for unhealthy alcohol use in primary care settings in adults 18 years or older, including pregnant women, and also recommends providing persons engaged in identified risky or hazardous drinking with brief behavioral counseling interventions.[2] Screeners can be easily and efficiently administered by the clinician or with a patient self-report form, and they can be used as an effective bridge to a more in-depth conversation about controlled substance prescription and nonprescription drug use when appropriate. It is important to remember that the goal of screening, whether by self-report form or by interview, is not to diagnose a substance use disorder

**Table 1**
**Evidence-based brief substance use screening tools**

| Tool/Link | Substance Type | How Administered |
|---|---|---|
| National Institute on Drug Abuse Drug Use Screening Tool: Quick Screen (NMASSIST) | Alcohol, tobacco, prescription medication, drugs | Self-administered or clinician-administered |
| CAGE Adapted to Include Drugs (CAGE-AID) | Alcohol, drugs | Clinician-administered |
| Brief Screener for Alcohol, Tobacco, and other Drugs (BSTAD) | Tobacco, alcohol, drugs | Self-administered or clinician-administered |
| Tobacco, Alcohol, Prescription medication, and other Substance use (TAPS) | Tobacco, alcohol, prescription medications | Self-administered or clinician-administered |

but rather to identify individuals who may be at elevated risk for problem alcohol, controlled substance, or recreational drug use. The screening process provides an important opportunity for the provider to conduct or recommend further risk assessment, brief counseling and referral, and/or clinical collaboration with other providers.

By definition, screening questionnaires are limited in scope, and a screener cannot elicit the breadth of information that can be collected through a well-executed face-to-face interview. This conclusion was supported in 2 early Dutch studies[3,4] that found that although self-report questionnaires may be more time-efficient than interview-based history-taking, combining questionnaire data with verbal history–taking represented a superior approach to information-gathering in the dental setting. For dental providers, the face-to-face history-taking interview is a key element of clinical care that not only serves to collect clinical data but also to establish a positive *therapeutic alliance* with the patient. In all areas of health care,[5–7] including dental medicine,[8,9] much has been written about the important role of the clinical interview in establishing the therapeutic alliance. Alliance building fosters trust and confidence in the clinician and is associated with greater patient satisfaction,[10] adherence with recommended therapies,[11] and better overall clinical outcomes.[12] The interrelationships among communication, trust, patient satisfaction, adherence, and outcomes have also been empirically supported in the dental literature.[13–16] Further, it has been demonstrated that effective patient interviewing leads to the collection of more clinically useful information from patients and helps facilitate patient-centered care through shared decision-making.[17] Demonstrable benefits of shared decision-making have been documented in both general[18,19] and dental[20,21] medicine literature.

## STRATEGIES FOR EFFECTIVE INTERVIEWING FOR RISK ASSESSMENT

A phenomenological approach to patient interviewing seeks to elicit and understand the patient's unique experience of his or her illness, demonstrates empathy, respects patient differences, and supports the individual's preferred communication style. This person-centered approach is widely supported across all fields of medicine and is also promoted in the pain management literature as superior for relationship building between patients and clinicians.[22] This approach is especially helpful to counter an unfortunate yet pervasive tendency for clinicians to disbelieve or dismiss patients' pain complaints.[23] The goal of the interview should be for the clinician to encourage and support an open, 2-way flow of information. Failure to effectively communicate may contribute to poorer outcomes, and dental or medical care that is not consistent with the patient's actual needs, values, and preferences.[24] Phenomenological inquiry has been encouraged in dental care as a means of creating honest and comprehensive exchanges between doctors and patients.[25,26]

Essential communication tasks in medical encounters have been defined by expert consensus[27] and these interview components together provide a useful framework for communication-oriented standards for all health professionals. Key interview strategies include the following:

- Building rapport and establishing a positive clinician-patient relationship
- Opening a 2-way discussion and establishing context for the clinical visit
- Gathering information and history-taking
- Asking questions to understand the patient's perspective on his or her illness
- Sharing information with the patient and providing appropriate patient education
- Reaching agreement on problems and plans
- Providing closure and defining next steps/follow-up care

Risk factor screening would typically be included in the "information-gathering" or history-taking phase of the clinical encounter. Because most patients will present with multiple risk factors, screening should be expanded to cover multiple risks[28] so as to minimize missed opportunities for identifying individuals who may benefit from brief intervention and referral and eliminate demographic disparities. Of course, patients may have significant concerns regarding sharing sensitive information pertaining to drug use, mental health symptoms, and domestic circumstances. Further, they may experience anxiety regarding confidentiality, embarrassment, and fear of being judged by the provider. These patient experiences may lead to failure to disclose important information regarding substance use patterns, resulting in a missed opportunity for referral for needed specialist care.[29]

When interviewing the dental patient regarding potentially sensitive or "taboo" topics (including substance use and mental health history), it is best practice to *contextualize and normalize* sensitive questions to ensure that the patient understands that there are legitimate clinical reasons for the inquiry. Normalizing helps dispel the notion that the patient is being "singled out" to provide details regarding sensitive topics. For example, the clinician may preface the conversation with: "To ensure the safest care possible, I ask all my patients about their alcohol and substance use; these may interact with anesthetics or with medications I might need to prescribe for your oral health problem." This statement can then be followed by an *open-ended question* such as, "Can you please tell me how many alcoholic drinks you have in a typical week?" Note that this question *presumes use of the substance*, thereby making it easier for the patient to respond in the affirmative if he or she uses (in any amount), whereas the abstinent patient can simply state "none."

Alternatively, a brief screener (such as the National Institute on Drug Abuse Quick Screen) could be administered as a starting point for the substance use history. The patient's responses should then be reviewed and details added with follow-up questions by the clinician or another trained member of the dental team. A screener provides an opportunity to ask individualized follow-up questions and, depending on the patient's responses, to advance to a conversation regarding the relationship between, tobacco, alcohol, or other substances and the patient's oral health risks. When it is made clear to the patient that the goal for substance use screening is to promote oral health and safe oral care, this contextualization promotes a positive and open conversation between patient and clinician. *Open-ended questions,* particularly in the early phases of the patient interview, are critical for effective data gathering. An open-ended question is one that prompts patients to describe or "tell their story," whereas a closed-ended question can be answered with a 1-word answer. Shifting interview style from primarily closed-ended questions ("What medicines do you take? Do you take your pain medication as prescribed?") to *empathic statements followed by an open-ended question* ("What you are describing sounds difficult. Can you tell me how you typically manage your pain?") will yield richer data while also strengthening the clinician's therapeutic alliance with the patient. Although one might assume that an open-ended style of questioning will take significantly more time, allowing patients a few minutes of uninterrupted time to express themselves reaps many rewards; not only will richer data be collected, but this approach demonstrates empathy and interest, essential elements for building trust in the clinician-patient relationship.

A controlled substance risk assessment interview should seek to identify potential risks in 3 separate yet related domains: substance use/misuse, mental health comorbidities, and pain conditions/pain management. All 3 areas may be directly or indirectly related to the patient's use of prescription and over-the-counter medications. A detailed medication history is critical and the interviewer should identify each medication used, the indication for its use, the dose and schedule, and the prescriber. Other important information that is too-often neglected is an assessment of the patient's adherence and, in the case of controlled substances, whether the patient is using the medication in ways for which it was not prescribed (misuse) or specifically for its psychoactive/euphorigenic effects (abuse). For any PRN (as-needed) drugs, the clinician should additionally inquire about dose and typical frequency of use. It is particularly important to use plain language when inquiring about medications and to include questions specifically regarding sleeping medications (sedative/hypnotics), pain medications, anxiety medications (benzodiazepines), or treatments for depression or other mental health conditions.

Interviewing the dental patient with a history of 1 or more chronic pain or mental health conditions may present a particular challenge for the dental provider, as these complex clinical issues unfortunately may be associated with negative stereotypes and concerns regarding "drug seeking" or medication misuse. As a result, the clinician may be uncomfortable addressing complex pain problems, compounding the patient's reluctance to disclose a pain diagnosis or treatment history for fear of being labeled as a "difficult patient." It is important for the dental clinician to become comfortable with routinely asking sensitive questions and responding with openness and empathy to the range of patient reactions to these sometimes-difficult conversations.

## ROLES OF DENTAL HYGIENISTS IN SUBSTANCE USE RISK ASSESSMENT AND INTERVENTION

Like other health care providers, dentists are often pressed for time[30,31] and may fear that engaging in open-ended patient dialogue regarding emotionally sensitive issues such as substance use will become too labor-intensive or time-intensive. Many clinicians perceive time constraints as a major barrier to the assessment of substance use, and this theme of insufficient time is well documented in the dental literature.[32–34] A provider in a recent qualitative study[35] stated, "So, I heard all this stuff that I'm supposed to be doing, taking a complete history, complete addiction history. . . But I don't have time to do what I am supposed to do in terms of proper treatment, opioid treatment, so I cut corners a bit" (p. 378). Rushing through the initial interview process has significant costs and restricts the collection of accurate information. To deal with issues of insufficient time in general medical settings, emphasis has been placed increasingly on expanding the role other members of the medical team to assess substance use risks.[36,37] A team-based approach is well suited to primary care settings, in which nonphysician providers typically spend more time in face-to-face interaction with patients than do physicians.[38,39] Similarly, dental hygienists and other members of the dental team may be a trained in substance use screening, brief intervention, and referral, with a small but growing body of literature supporting this approach.

Dental hygiene education, even more than dental education, places a strong emphasis on preventive strategies that support oral health and overall health. It has been demonstrated that dental hygiene visits are often scheduled more consistently and that these visits are also of longer duration[40] than primary care visits, presenting an important opportunity to incorporate substance screening into the context of dental care. In one comparative study of health professions students regarding their attitudes and beliefs about tobacco cessation counseling, only dental hygiene students were in 100% agreement that they were adequately prepared to help patients with this health-related behavior.[41] This finding is likely associated with the 2004 inclusion of a requirement for training in tobacco cessation[42] by the American Dental Association

Accreditation Standards for Dental Hygiene Programs. In an article by Gordon and Severson[40] regarding barriers to providing tobacco cessation counseling, the investigators' first recommendation was for the dental hygienist to be designated as the lead member of the oral health team with regard to behavioral interventions for nicotine addiction. Because most dental insurances do not yet cover tobacco cessation counseling, it might also be cost-effective to train other members of the dental team to include substance use screening along with other health history review, rather than focus exclusively on dentists to provide this important intervention.

Dental hygienists are already well-trained to explore and address nicotine addiction in the primary dental care setting, and the training and role of the dental hygiene practitioner could be easily expanded to include screening and brief intervention regarding the use of other substances. In a 2015 study regarding the effectiveness of screening and brief intervention for alcohol abuse in dental practice,[43] the investigators noted the dental hygienists' high level of skill for rapport-building with patients and encouraging open discussions through the use of open-ended questions. As in other studies, the investigators noted that the ratio of dental hygienists to dentists makes them the obvious dental health professionals for initiating such protocols. Although little has been written on dental hygienists' roles regarding actual counseling for alcohol and illicit drugs, an article by Boyer and colleagues[44] noted that dental hygienists could play an active role in screening adolescent users of methamphetamine. Given adolescents' developmentally appropriate concerns with appearance and peer acceptance, conversations regarding risks of methamphetamine use (including "meth mouth") have the potential to impact adolescents' future drug use. The oral effects of methamphetamine use are well known and stigmatizing for many users,[45] so open and nonjudgmental discussions using a motivational interviewing approach (see the article on motivational interviewing by Schatman et al, elsewhere in this issue) has the potential to impact substance use behaviors.

Substance use screening has other applications for hygiene practice, including risk assessment before opioid prescribing. Although not widely known, dental hygienists have opioid prescribing authority in 4 states: Colorado, Maine, New Mexico, and Oregon.[46] Hygienists who prescribe opioids have an ethical and legal obligation to do so safely; rapport-building, open communication, and assessing risks of administration of opioids goes hand-in-hand with the prescribing of controlled substances. In an article on psychosocial opioid risk assessment in orofacial pain,[47] the investigators noted that screening questionnaires are generally insufficient for assessing risk, and recommended an interactive discussion between the clinician and the patient.

There has been a strong movement over the past several years to replace the routine prescribing of opioids with nonopioid medications for dental procedures. Numerous studies have found that alternate pain management strategies[48,49] are safe and effective, but the limited use of opioids will remain clinically necessary for some patients. Further, some individuals who present for dental care will be taking opioid medications and other controlled substances for nondental indications. Dentists, dental hygienists, and other members of the dental team are well positioned to help mitigate opioid risk through effective communication, screening, and risk assessment to ensure safe and appropriate analgesia by thoroughly exploring all relevant risk factors prior to prescribing controlled substances.

## SUMMARY

In their broadly defined roles as health care providers, dentists, like all clinicians, require patient-centered communication skills to obtain accurate clinical information regarding potential substance use, misuse, and abuse, as well as related issues of mental health comorbidities and pain conditions. Using these skills will ensure holistic and likely more effective treatment. Controlled substance, alcohol, and recreational drug use not only has overall health implications, but also clear connections to oral health risks and the safe practice of dental medicine. Despite the temptation to rely solely on self-report questionnaires in the name of expedience, the face-to-face clinical interview remains the most effective way of establishing a therapeutic alliance and for collecting clinical data relevant to substance use risk. Patient-centered interviewing approaches that acknowledge and validate the patient's unique life experiences strengthen the clinician-patient relationship, foster positive communication, and help overcome barriers to adherence to recommended care plans. All members of the dental team should be educated and encouraged to engage in open, respectful, and empathic dialogue with patients to collect critical information regarding substance use to ensure safe and effective dental care. We have recommended patient-centered approaches to interviewing dental patients that are consistent with primary care and pain literature and will help the dentist to identify potential substance use risks early in treatment. Applying this approach will facilitate an open exchange between the dental provider and the patient, demonstrate respect for the patient's unique life world, and minimize the risk of alienation and diminished patient engagement while fostering empathy for the patient. We have also argued for an expanded role of the dental hygienist as a cost-efficient approach to substance use screening and brief intervention. As dental hygienists are skilled in tobacco cessation counseling, we suggest that dental hygienists' roles can be expanded to screen and provide brief counseling for patients who may be at risk of substance use problems. This expanded role in no way diminishes the role that dentists need to play in risk assessment, but rather highlights that a team-based approach to building greater capacity for risk assessment and safer prescribing will ultimately lead to improved outcomes.

## ACKNOWLEDGMENT

This work was funded in part by a grant from the Coverys Community Healthcare Foundation.

## DISCLOSURE

The authors have nothing to disclose.

## REFERENCES

1. Hölund U, Theilade E, Poulsen S. Validity of a dietary interviewing method for use in caries prevention. Community Dent Oral Epidemiol 1985;13(4):219–21.

2. US Preventive Services Task Force. Screening and behavioral counseling interventions to reduce unhealthy alcohol use in adolescents and adults: US preventive services task force recommendation statement. JAMA 2018;320(18): 1899–909.

3. de Jong KJ, Abraham-Inpijn L, Oomen HA, et al. Clinical relevance of a medical history in dental practice: comparison between a questionnaire and a dialogue. Community Dent Oral Epidemiol 1991;19(5):310–1.

4. de Jong KJ, Borgmeijer-Hoelen A, Abraham-Inpijn L. Validity of a risk-related patient-administered medical questionnaire for dental patients. Oral Surg Oral Med Oral Pathol 1991;72(5):527–33.

5. Brown RT, Henderson PB. Treating the adolescent: the initial meeting. Semin Adolesc Med 1987;3(2):79–91.
6. Rossi L, Leary E. Evaluating the patient with coronary artery disease. Nurs Clin North Am 1992;27(1):171–88.
7. Hilsenroth MJ, Cromer TD. Clinician interventions related to alliance during the initial interview and psychological assessment. Psychotherapy (Chic) 2007; 44(2):205–18.
8. Epstein S. Treatment of the geriatric dentally phobic patient. Dent Clin North Am 1988;32(4):715–21.
9. Antoniadou M, Kitopoulou A, Kapsalas A, et al. Basic tips for communicating with a new dental patient. ARC Dent Sci 2016;1(4):4–11.
10. Georgopoulou S, Prothero L, D'Cruz DP. Physician-patient communication in rheumatology: a systematic review. Rheumatol Int 2018;38(5):763–75.
11. Pereira MG, Pedras S, Ferreira G, et al. Differences, predictors, and moderators of therapeutic adherence in patients recently diagnosed with type 2 diabetes. J Health Psychol 2018. [Epub ahead of print].
12. Lee YY, Lin JL. The effects of trust in physician on self-efficacy, adherence and diabetes outcomes. Soc Sci Med 2009;68(6):1060–8.
13. Dyer TA, Owens J, Robinson PG. What matters to patients when their care is delegated to dental therapists? Br Dent J 2013;214(6):E17.
14. Wong L, Ryan FS, Christensen LR, et al. Factors influencing satisfaction with the process of orthodontic treatment in adult patients. Am J Orthod Dentofacial Orthop 2018;153(3):362–70.
15. Badri P, Saltaji H, Flores-Mir C, et al. Factors affecting children's adherence to regular dental attendance: a systematic review. J Am Dent Assoc 2014;145(8): 817–28.
16. Carey JA, Madill A, Manogue M. Communications skills in dental education: a systematic research review. Eur J Dent Educ 2010;14(2):69–78.
17. Kaplan SH, Greenfield S, Gandek B, et al. Characteristics of physicians with participatory decision-making styles. Ann Intern Med 1996;124(5):497–504.
18. Brown L, Gardner G, Bonner A. A randomized controlled trial testing a decision support intervention for older patients with advanced kidney disease. J Adv Nurs 2019;75(11):3032–44.
19. Wilson SR, Strub P, Buist AS, et al. Shared treatment decision making improves adherence and outcomes in poorly controlled asthma. Am J Respir Crit Care Med 2010;181(6):566-577.
20. Bauer J, Spackman S, Chiappelli F, et al. Model of evidence-based dental decision making. J Evid Based Dent Pract 2005;5(4):189–97.
21. Ghaeminia H, Perry J, Nienhuijs ME, et al. Surgical removal versus retention for the management of asymptomatic disease-free impacted wisdom teeth. Cochrane Database Syst Rev 2016;(8):CD003879.
22. Chen AT, Swaminathan A. Factors in the building of effective patient-provider relationships in the context of fibromyalgia. Pain Med 2019;21(1):138–49.
23. Ojala T, Häkkinen A, Karppinen J, et al. Although unseen, chronic pain is real: a phenomenological study. Scand J Pain 2015;6(1):33–40.
24. Stenner R, Palmer S, Hammond R. What matters most to people in musculoskeletal physiotherapy consultations? A qualitative study. Musculoskelet Sci Pract 2018;35:84–9.
25. Bowers JA, Wilson JE. Graduates' perceptions of self-assessment training in clinical dental hygiene education. J Dent Educ 2002;66(10):1146–53.

26. Bernson JM, Hallberg LR, Elfström ML, et al. Making dental care possible: a mutual affair': a grounded theory relating to adult patients with dental fear and regular dental treatment. Eur J Oral Sci 2011;119(5):373–80.
27. Makoul G. Essential elements of communication in medical encounters: the Kalamazoo consensus statement. Acad Med 2001;76(4):390–3.
28. Coups EJ, Gaba A, Orleans CT. Physician screening for multiple behavioral health risk factors. Am J Prev Med 2004;27(2 Suppl):34–41.
29. Sankar P, Jones NL. To tell or not to tell primary care patients' disclosure deliberations. Arch Intern Med 2005;165(20):2378–83.
30. Turner JA, Dworkin SF. Screening for psychosocial risk factors in patients with chronic orofacial pain: recent advances. J Am Dent Assoc 2004;135(8):1119–25.
31. Carrilho E, Dianiskova S, Guncu GN, et al. Practical implementation of evidence-based dentistry into daily dental practice through a short time dependent searching method. J Evid Based Dent Pract 2016;16(1):7–18.
32. McNeely J, Wright S, Matthews AG, et al. Substance-use screening and interventions in dental practices: survey of practice-based research network dentists regarding current practices, policies and barriers. J Am Dent Assoc 2013; 144(6):627–38.
33. Rush WA, Schleyer TK, Kirshner M, et al. Integrating tobacco dependence counseling into electronic dental records: a multi-method approach. J Dent Educ 2014;78(1):31–9.
34. Satterwhite S, Knight KR, Miaskowski C, et al. Sources and impact of time pressure on opioid management in the safety-net. J Am Board Fam Med 2019;32(3): 375–82.
35. Norberg MM, Gates P, Dillon P, et al. Screening and managing cannabis use: comparing GP's and nurses' knowledge, beliefs, and behavior. Subst Abuse Treat Prev Policy 2012;7:31.
36. Wamsley M, Satterfield JM, Curtis A, et al. Alcohol and drug screening, brief intervention, and referral to treatment (SBIRT) training and implementation: perspectives from 4 health professions. J Addict Med 2018;12(4):262–72.
37. Laurant M, van der Biezen M, Wijers N, et al. Nurses as substitutes for doctors in primary care. Cochrane Database Syst Rev 2018;(7):CD001271.
38. Lockwood C. Nurses as substitutes for doctors in primary care: a Cochrane review summary. Int J Nurs Stud 2019. [Epub ahead of print].
39. Gordon JS, Albert DA, Crews KM, et al. Tobacco education in dentistry and dental hygiene. Drug Alcohol Rev 2009;28(5):517–32.
40. Gordon JS, Severson HH. Tobacco cessation through dental office settings. J Dent Educ 2001;65:354–63.
41. Fried JL, Reid BC, DeVore LE. A comparison of health professions student attitudes regarding tobacco curricula and interventionist roles. J Dent Educ 2004; 68(3):370–7.
42. American Dental Education Association. Exhibit 5: ADEA policy statements. J Dent Educ 2004;68(7):729–44.
43. Neff JA, Kelley ML, Walters ST, et al. Effectiveness of a Screening and Brief Intervention protocol for heavy drinkers in dental practice: a cluster-randomized trial. J Health Psychol 2015;20(12):1534–48.
44. Boyer EM, Thompson N, Hill T, et al. The relationship between methamphetamine use and dental caries and missing teeth. J Dent Hyg 2015;89(2):119–31.
45. Murphy DA, Harrell L, Fintzy R, et al. A comparison of methamphetamine users to a matched NHANES cohort: propensity score analyses for oral health care and dental service need. J Behav Health Serv Res 2016;43(4):676–90.

46. Lutfiyya MN, Gross AJ, Schvaneveldt N, et al. A scoping review exploring the opioid prescribing practices of US dental professionals. J Am Dent Assoc 2018;149(12):1011–23.

47. Kulich RJ, Backstrom J, Brownstein J, et al. A model for opioid risk stratification: assessing the psychosocial components of orofacial pain. Oral Maxillofac Surg Clin North Am 2016;28(3):261–73.

48. Chakote K, Guggenheimer J. Implications of use of opioid-containing analgesics for palliation of acute dental pain. J Opioid Manag 2019;15(1):35–41.

49. Wang TT, Hersh EV, Panchal N. Covering the prescription drug monitoring program gap: using shared decision making to reduce dental opioid prescriptions. J Oral Maxillofac Surg 2019;77(1):7–8.

# Special Screening Resources

## Strategies to Identify Substance Use Disorders, Including Opioid Misuse and Abuse

David A. Keith, BDS, FDSRCS, DMD[a],*,
María F. Hernández-Nuño de la Rosa, DDS, MS[b]

### KEYWORDS

- Dentistry • Pain • Substance use disorder • Opioid risk tool • NIDA quick screen
- Interprofessional collaboration

### KEY POINTS

- Dentists should use screening tools (eg, Opioid Risk Tool and NIDA Quick Screen) and other techniques to identify patients at risk for developing SUD and be able to intervene upon suspicion or identification of an SUD.
- Dentists should identify the rationale for and benefits of active communication and collaboration with other treating clinicians (interprofessional collaboration) and know when to consult with a Pain specialist.
- Dentists should recognize the importance of periodic reassessment, follow-up, and documentation with ongoing and long-term management of pain and opioid analgesics.

## INTRODUCTION

The prescription drug crisis has affected all sectors of the population, and so it is inevitable that dentists will increasingly see at-risk patients or those with substance use disorders (SUD) in the course of their professional activities. Recognizing these patients and the special needs that they may have is now part of the standard of care for the profession. Screening for substance misuse involves a thorough history and review of the patient's medical record and, as appropriate, reviewing prior records. Several risk assessment tools are available that can help identify relevant risk factors and quantify the level of substance misuse risk. Accessing the patients' prescription drug monitoring program (PDMP) data will identify the recent history of controlled substance prescriptions and provide information on potential misuse activities. None of

[a] Department of Oral and Maxillofacial Surgery, Massachusetts General Hospital, Warren 1201, Fruit Street, Boston, MA 02114, USA; [b] Craniofacial Pain Center, Department of Diagnostic Sciences, Tufts University School of Dental Medicine, 1 Kneeland Street, Boston, MA 02111, USA
* Corresponding author.
E-mail address: DKeith@partners.org

Dent Clin N Am 64 (2020) 513–524
https://doi.org/10.1016/j.cden.2020.03.002
0011-8532/20/© 2020 Elsevier Inc. All rights reserved.

these tools are definitive but can help to provide information to the dentist in order to identify and discuss risk factors with the patient.

## PRESCRIPTION DRUG MONITORING PROGRAMS

PDMPs are state-run programs that collect and distribute data about the prescription of controlled substances.[1] These programs are administered by a variety of state agencies, including Boards of Pharmacy, Departments of Health, Professional Licensing Boards, and Law Enforcement Agencies. The intent of PDMPs is to help prevent substance misuse by providing historic data on patient's-controlled substance prescriptions. All states, other than Missouri, currently have a PDMP in effect, and many state programs are interoperable with those in other states (**Fig. 1**).[2] The goal is to have all state-based PDMPs interoperable, so prescribers can check their patients'-controlled substance history across the country.

As an example, the Massachusetts PDMP, administered by the Department of Public Health and now called Massachusetts Prescription Awareness Tool (MassPAT), is a computer-based system that collects controlled substance prescription data submitted by pharmacies in the state and those who deliver controlled substances medications to the state on all controlled substances, within 1 business day. In Massachusetts, this includes all opioids, benzodiazepines, gabapentin, and tramadol. The data provide registered users, including dentists with the appropriate licenses, with information about the controlled substance prescription data for their patients.

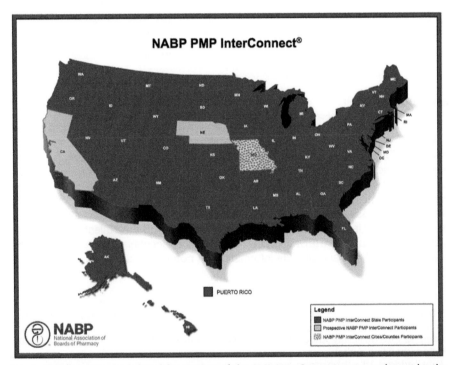

**Fig. 1.** PDMPs interoperability. (The version of the PMP InterConnect map used must be the current PDF published to the NABP website at https://nabp.pharmacy/wp-content/uploads/2019/04/PMP-InterConnect-Map-August-2019.pdf. Reprinted with permission: National Association of Boards of Pharmacy® (NABP®), Mount Prospect, IL.)

Each state has its own specific regulations, and in Massachusetts, use of the database has been mandated since October 2016. The law instructs prescribers to check this database each time when prescribing controlled substances.[3] PDMP data can indicate forged and altered prescriptions, doctor shopping, prescription rings, unlawful dispensing, as well as prescription, distribution, and health care fraud. Data show that there is a greater impact on clinician adherence with this mandate in place.[4]

## PRESCRIPTION MONITORING PROGRAM DATA

The MassPAT database consists of the patient's name, date of birth, sex, address, name of the drugs prescribed, strength, quantity, number of days, prescriber name, prescription number, pharmacy where filled, number of refills, morphine equivalency per day (morphine milligram equivalents [MME]), payment type, and state where prescription was filled. It also lists the prescribers' names, addresses, and telephone numbers, as well as the pharmacies' name, address, and telephone number. A summary provides the total number of controlled prescriptions, number of prescribers, pharmacies used, private pay numbers, and active daily MME in the last year. Each of these pieces of data can be useful and is subject to interpretation.

- *Name.* Patients may be known by nicknames or abbreviated names but are listed in the database under their legal names, sometimes with a middle initial (eg, Jackie Smith vs Jacqueline Smith vs Jacqueline M. Smith). Misspellings are also possible.
- *Date of birth* is a mandatory field and will differentiate between people with the same name but different birth dates.
- *Address.* Addresses can be entered with varying information (ie, apartment numbers, street names, and local community names vs municipality [Charlestown vs Boston, MA]). Two addresses may indicate that the person has moved but can also show that the person is registered at 2 or more separate locations, sometimes with the intent to escape detection. This is less likely now with increased interoperability.
- *Medications listed.* Each US state defines which medications are listed, and these lists are updated from time to time (eg, Massachusetts added gabapentin [Neurontin] to its list of reported medications in August 2017). Generally, opioids and benzodiazepines are listed. A combination of opioids with benzodiazepines is a sign of concern because 71% of prescription drug overdoses involve opioids and 31% involve benzodiazepines.[5]
- *Quantity and days prescribed* allow a calculation of number of doses per day. This helps with identification of overlapping prescriptions or early refills. Medications prescribed within a formal methadone maintenance program are not listed in MassPAT; other states also have some limitations on the drugs that are listed.
- *Prescribers.* Multiple prescribers for the same or similar medications could indicate "doctor shopping," which is one of the primary ways that people obtain prescription drugs for nonmedical use. However, considering the organization of the health care system, numerous prescribers may not represent a problem because several individuals listed at the same address may represent physicians and nurse practitioners working in the same facility all with access to the same medical record.
- *Pharmacies.* The number of different pharmacies a patient uses may be a cause of concern. Patients may legitimately use pharmacies close to home or to work for convenience or several pharmacies within the same chain.

- *A combination of multiple prescribers and multiple pharmacies.* Multiple pre-scribers and multiple pharmacies combined can indicate misuse potential. There is no universal definition, but 5 prescribers in any 1 year and 4 pharmacies in any 90-day period is used by MassPAT to indicate a level of concern and to generate reports for prescribers to alert them to potential issues.
- *Mean morphine equivalency.* Opinions vary as to the definition of "high dosing." The Centers for Disease Control and Prevention suggest that there is a need to address risk at more than MME of 50 mgm/d and encourages clinicians to avoid risk at greater than MME of 90 mgm/d[6] Dunn and colleagues[7] have stated that more than an MME of 100 mgm/d resulted in an 8.8-fold increase in overdose risk. Most dental surgery patients requiring opioids will have an MME of 50 mgm/d or less.
- *Payment type.* The cost of controlled substances for legitimate purposes is usu-ally covered under medical insurance, with copayments or limitations of quantity, and time between refills mandated by the state or insurance carrier. Self-pay may suggest that the patient is avoiding these restrictions.

The Massachusetts Department of Public Health added the Visano Opioid Steward-ship Platform to the MassPAT system on December 9, 2019. This system offers a rep-resentation of the data in an interactive form, allowing prescribers and pharmacists to more quickly and easily understand the data and help improve clinical decision mak-ing and patient safety. It also provides tools and resources for patients. The system supplements the data found in the MassPAT database: in addition, patient demo-graphics and risk indicators are displayed, and prescribing history is shown in graphic form in addition to a list of local SUD treatment resources. The summary and prescrip-tion data are the same as the original MassPAT data. Risk indicators, chosen by Mass-PAT, include "More than 5 providers in any year (365 Days), More than 4 pharmacies in any 90-day period and more than 40 MME/day and more than 100 MME total."[8]

## TYPES OF MISUSE

- *Doctor shopping.* It implies that the patient is going from 1 physician's or den-tist's office to another and obtaining multiple prescriptions for opioids or other controlled substances for the same symptom. Individual states' PDMPs classify such cases as "activities of concern" because more detail is often needed before assuming illegal behavior. This behavior is typically characterized by the patient having multiple pill bottles labeled for the same opioid medication, prescribed by multiple practitioners, and frequently filled at multiple pharmacies to avoid detec-tion. The typical scenario is for the patient to present with factitious symptoms, and once an opioid prescription has been obtained, move on to the next location. Dentists are particularly at risk because they predominantly practice alone or in small groups and do not have ready access to patients' medical records or to colleagues practicing nearby. This scam can also be perpetrated on several members of a group practice especially if they have more than 1 office location and do not have a robust and timely way to communicate repeat appointments, multiple medications, and outside-of-business-hours' refill requests. This type of activity has been difficult to detect without the real-time data provided by the PDMP. This behavior was documented in a 2017 National Public Radio segment in which 2 prior opioid abusers in a recovery program described how they main-tained broken teeth in their mouths to get dentists to prescribe opioids.[9] Accord-ing to Massachusetts law, patients have the responsibility of informing their providers if they are being treated by another provider and receiving prescriptions for the same ailment. Providers can also refuse to write a prescription if they feel the patient is not being truthful. Doctor shopping and other drug-seeking behaviors point to the benefit of health care professionals' using tools[10] to help assess opioid addiction risk.

- *Hoarding.* In anticipation of increased pain related to upcoming surgery, patients can mislead their providers about the number of opioid pills they are taking with the result that they hoard medications for an anticipated increased need or "for a rainy day." Such behavior also heightens the risk of death by suicide or unintended overdose.
- *Diversion.* It occurs when legally produced controlled pharmaceuticals are illegally obtained for nonmedical use. Examples include physicians, dentists, or pharmacists selling prescriptions or drugs to nonpatients, employee theft, doctor shopping, robberies, and prescription forgeries. Cases of veterinary opioid pain medications being diverted to the human population have been reported.
- *Overlapping prescriptions.* This is a form of misuse that can occur in different ways. The patient can request early refills from the primary provider or go to another provider for a duplicate prescription. The frequent excuses are vacation requests, increased use due to special circumstances (for example, stressful unforeseen circumstances, trauma, weather changes), and so forth. Patients can also acquire prescriptions for overlapping medical or surgical conditions; for example, a dental extraction while receiving treatment for an orthopedic injury.

Utilization of PDMP data is just 1 way that clinicians can assess the risk for patients who may experience substance misuse.[11] Risk assessment tools, such as the National Institute on Drug Abuse quick screen[12] and Opioid Risk Tool,[10] together with a careful history, accurate diagnosis, and pain management plan are essential elements for ensuring that patients have their pain controlled in an appropriate and safe manner.

The impact of PDMPs as an opioid risk management tool is mixed. The data can help avoid "doctor shopping" and drug interactions. It is also helpful in communication between prescribers and interactions with patients. Concern has been expressed that the data can have a "chilling effect" on prescribing habits and lead to undertreatment of pain and the cause of patients turning to illicit drugs.[13] Rasubala and colleagues[14] found that the impact of mandatory PDMPs significantly reduced the number of opioid prescriptions and number of pills prescribed by dentists.

In Massachusetts, over the period CY2015 to CY2018, controlled substance prescriptions decreased for "all prescribers" and for "all dentists" and continued to decrease after the MassPAT program went live on August 22, 2016. Searches by dentists increased dramatically in the quarter before implementation until October 15, 2016 when all prescribers were required to check the database before prescribing opioids; thereafter, the number of searches remained constant. During this timeframe, prescription counts dropped 47% (60% nationally); solid quantity dropped 55%; and total MME/day dropped 58%. Days' supply per patient was reduced by 16%, and 20% of prescribers did not renew their prescribing licenses. Dentists also prescribed alternative medications for pain control nationally, 34%, and in Massachusetts, 39%.[14-17]

The Massachusetts Department of Public Health has recently launched The Massachusetts Substance Use Helpline, a free tool for finding substance use treatment and recovery services. It also provides overdose education, including naloxone distribution sites.[18] In addition, a mobile application is now available to help health care providers apply the recommendations of the Centers for Disease Control and Prevention's Guideline for Prescribing Opioids for Chronic Pain into the clinical setting.[19] This application includes a Total Daily Opioid Dose (MME) Calculator to identify more quickly patients at risk of overdose as well as access to prescribing guidance and information on motivational interviewing to improve the decision-making process and the communication skills, respectively. All these resources are helpful for the dentist, who may not be part of a broader health care team.

## OPIOID RISK ASSESSMENT

In a recent study, 58% of Massachusetts dentists thought assessment of substance use was within their scope of practice, with 95% registering with MassPAT. However, the compliance rate was only 20% compared with physicians at 60%. Nationally, 50% of dentists stated that they assessed PDMPs,[20] and in Massachusetts, the number was 38% (5% consistently). Ten percent of Massachusetts dentists used forms or questionnaires to assess opioid risk, and 76% "asked patients directly." The ability to assess risk was related to levels of training.[21]

## SCREENING TOOLS

Massachusetts law requires that prescribers assess risk before prescribing opioids, and several instruments are available. The National Institute on Drug Abuse (NIDA) Quick Screen (**Figs. 2 and 3**) asks "how often you have used alcohol, tobacco products, prescription drugs for non-medical purposes and illegal drugs in the past year." This app can be used on a smart phone and administered in a few minutes; the risk score is calculated and displayed once the information has been entered. The Opioid

**National Institute on Drug Abuse Quick Screen**

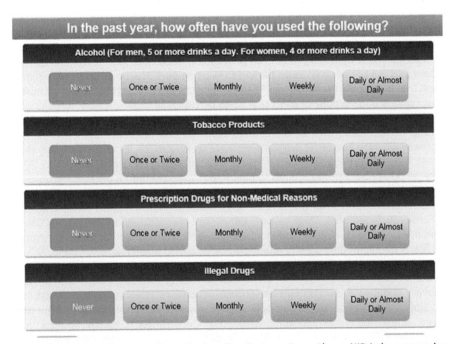

**Fig. 2.** The NIDA quick screen. (*From* National Institute on Drug Abuse. NIDA drug screening tool. Available at: https://www.drugabuse.gov/nmassist/.)

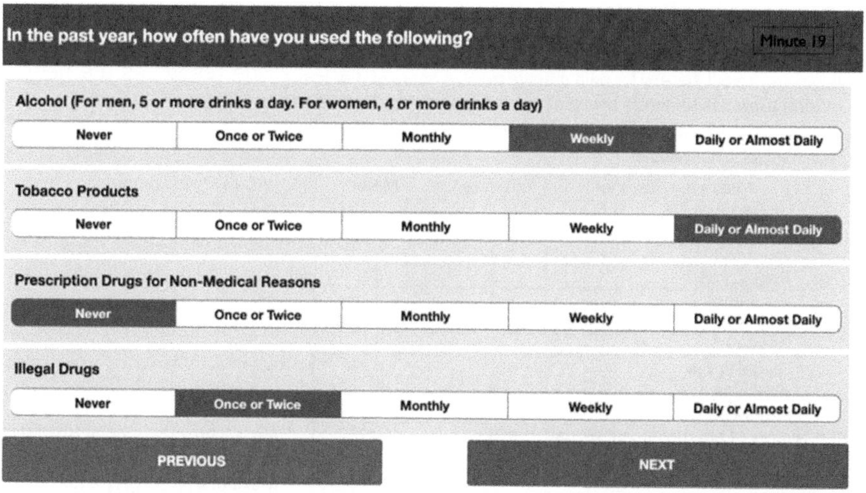

**In the past year, how often have you used the following?**    Minute 19

Alcohol (For men, 5 or more drinks a day. For women, 4 or more drinks a day)

| Never | Once or Twice | Monthly | Weekly | Daily or Almost Daily |

Tobacco Products

| Never | Once or Twice | Monthly | Weekly | Daily or Almost Daily |

Prescription Drugs for Non-Medical Reasons

| Never | Once or Twice | Monthly | Weekly | Daily or Almost Daily |

Illegal Drugs

| Never | Once or Twice | Monthly | Weekly | Daily or Almost Daily |

PREVIOUS          NEXT

**Fig. 3.** The NIDA quick screen: National Institute on Drug Abuse Quick Screen example. (*From* National Institute on Drug Abuse. NIDA drug screening tool. Available at: https://www.drugabuse.gov/nmassist/.)

Risk Tool (**Figs. 4 and 5**) asks the same questions with the addition of asking about a history of sexual abuse in preteenage years for women, a factor that is highly associated with opioid abuse in later life.[10] Each positive response is scored, and low risk is graded at lower than 3, medium risk 4 to 7, and high risk 8 or above.

## CASE HISTORIES

Six case histories will give examples of the type of information that PDMPs and screening tools can provide and how the information can be used in the management of the patient's pain.

1 *Dentist shopping.* A 33-year-old health care worker who had recently moved from a neighboring state presents to a dentist's office with "jaw pain." The history and examination are not consistent with the patient's complaints. She requested an opioid prescription, which the dentist declined. A check of her PDMP demonstrated that in the past 6 months she had filled 20 controlled prescriptions: 16 opioids and 2 benzodiazepines from 10 prescribers (15 were dentists practicing in a large metropolitan area). She had used 10 pharmacies and had a similar profile from the neighboring state. This pattern represents "shopping" for controlled substances by visiting dental offices and faking symptoms with the expectation that the dentists would not communicate with each other.

2 *Substance abuse.* A 49-year-old woman had undergone prior temporomandibular joint (TMD) surgery and presented with recurrent temporomandibular joint pain. She requested opioid prescriptions because her "other doctors had referred her with enough pills until this appointment." A review of her PDMP revealed that she was registered under 2 names at 2 locations. In the past year, she had had 151 controlled substance prescriptions: 97 opioids, 20 benzodiazepines, and 19 anxiolytics. These had been prescribed by 53 unique prescribers, 10 of whom were dentists, and filled at 27 pharmacies. In confronting the patient with this information, she became angry and threatened to sue the state and the dentist for possessing this information. After reviewing a

### Opioid Risk Tool

This tool should be administered to patients upon an initial visit prior to beginning opioid therapy for pain management. A score of 3 or lower indicates low risk for future opioid abuse, a score of 4 to 7 indicates moderate risk for opioid abuse, and a score of 8 or higher indicates a high risk for opioid abuse.

| Mark each box that applies | Female | Male |
|---|---|---|
| Family history of substance abuse | | |
| Alcohol | 1 | 3 |
| Illegal drugs | 2 | 3 |
| Rx drugs | 4 | 4 |
| Personal history of substance abuse | | |
| Alcohol | 3 | 3 |
| Illegal drugs | 4 | 4 |
| Rx drugs | 5 | 5 |
| Age between 16–45y | 1 | 1 |
| History of preadolescent sexual abuse | 3 | 0 |
| Psychological Disease | | |
| ADD, OCD, bipolar, schizophrenia | 2 | 2 |
| Depression | 1 | 1 |
| Scoring totals | | |

Massachusetts General Hospital Department of Oral and Maxillofacial Surgery and Orofacial pain group Intake form

**Fig. 4.** The opioid risk tool.

few of these prescriptions with her, she settled down and agreed to the dentist calling her primary care physician (PCP) for a referral to a substance abuse program. Two years later, the patient returned with TMD pain; a review of her current MassPAT data showed that she was in an SUD program and taking suboxone. During this period, she had visited one of her original dentists, who had given her 2 prescriptions for

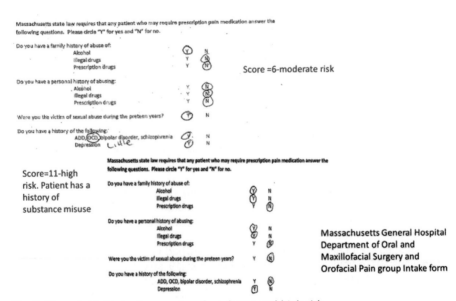

**Fig. 5.** The opioid risk tool: examples of moderate and high risk.

oxycodone. Did this dentist recognize her prescription drug misuse, and did they consult with her addiction specialist about prescribing an opioid?

3 *Appropriate chronic pain management.* A 35-year-old woman status post multiple facial traumas from a motor vehicle accident requiring reconstructive surgery presented. She continued to complain of pain, which was diagnosed as myofascial and neurogenic in origin. She is maintained on monthly prescriptions of opioid and benzodiazepines by an orofacial pain dentist who monitors pain and compliance. She uses 2 pharmacies and 2 prescribers within the same practice. This is an appropriate management of chronic pain.

4 *Recent questionable activity.* A 37-year-old woman with chronic pain is being seen on a regular 28-day cycle for prescription of 0.5 tablet of 10 mgm oxycodone/acetaminophen twice a day. She has an opioid contract on file. A follow-up review of her PDMP shows that in the past 2 months she has had additional prescriptions for 2- to 3-day-supply of opioids from 3 other physicians filled at multiple pharmacies other than her regular one. She denies knowledge of these other prescriptions. Is this doctor shopping, divergence, misuse, impersonation, or a reporting error? What should the dentist do? Because the patient denies that she ever filled these prescriptions, a check can be made to the pharmacies and physicians to verify the prescriptions. After the patient was informed that this would occur, she did not return to the practice.

5 *Prescriptions for overlapping medical conditions.* A 56-year-old nurse on long-term opioid therapy for muscle pain consisting of 2.5 mg oxycodone twice a day was seen. She had recently had orthopedic surgery requiring additional opioids and had recently been diagnosed with breast cancer. She had a lumpectomy and was given opioids by her surgeon. She underwent radiation therapy and suffered complications requiring higher-dose opioids from her oncologist. She presents to her dentist for the surgical removal of a tooth and requested a further prescription of opioids postoperatively. What should the dentist do? The dentist should request that either the PCP be the sole prescriber of pain medications or that she be referred to a pain management program and find alternative nonopioid medications for her postoperative pain. All other prescribers should be informed.

6 *Using opioids for other purposes.* A 69-year-old woman with long-term complaints of burning mouth syndrome and toothache had been prescribed a combination of opioids and benzodiazepines. In the past year, she had had 49 prescriptions: 24 opioids, 25 benzodiazepines from 7 prescribers and 2 pharmacies. She and her husband had their medical care through a clinic embedded in his institution where she saw numerous physicians within the same medical practice, and the prescriptions were filled at their local pharmacy or at the institutional pharmacy where the husband works. Her pain complaints were unrelieved by the medications. She was referred to a Pain specialist within a Pain Management Program who evaluated her and thought that she was using these medications to mitigate her other symptoms of depression, anxiety, and sleep disorders and was not addicted. She was slowly weaned off both prescriptions. Her symptoms were unchanged.

## LIABILITY

The issue of liability for using or not using the PDMP databases has not been clearly defined and depends on the current laws of the state. The prescribing dentist has a duty of care to the patient to warn them about the adverse effects of the medications prescribed and to act with reasonable care and in good faith when prescribing medications for pain control.[22,23]

## INTERVENTION UPON SUSPICION OF A SUBSTANCE USE DISORDER

Once the patient's risks of prescription opioid misuse have been assessed and issues of concern have been identified, the question becomes how to use this information in providing safe and appropriate clinical care. The decision tree can be divided into 3 domains[24]:

- *The primary prevention domain.* For a patient who is at low risk, the clinician evaluates the patient's pain and risk of substance misuse, prescribes pharmacologic treatment, and recommends nonpharmacologic treatment. The risks and benefits of the various modalities are discussed and, for controlled substances, appropriate storage and disposal instructions are given.
- *The secondary prevention domain.* When patients are determined to be at risk for SUD, the clinician should engage the patients in safe, informed, and patient-centered treatment planning. The clinician should have the ability to appropriately refer patients to pain management specialists. The clinician should provide special attention to safe prescribing and recognizing patients displaying signs of aberrant prescription use behaviors. Consultation with the patient's PCP or other providers may be necessary.
- *The tertiary prevention domain.* The clinician should view managing SUD as a chronic disease, thereby eliminating the stigma of addiction. The clinician should foster interdisciplinary and interprofessional collaborative efforts to reduce substance misuse. Managing acute pain in a patient with a SUD requires close collaboration with the patient's pain management team.

## LONG-TERM MANAGEMENT OF CHRONIC OROFACIAL PAIN

Clinicians who elect to follow patients over the long term should be prepared to constantly reassess the patient's diagnoses, treatment plan, and responses to treatment. Periodic second opinions are valuable in assuring that treatment goals are being met. Constant surveillance for signs of misuse is obligatory, and referral to a Pain specialist for continuing care is frequently a preferred option in the dental setting.

## DISCLOSURE

The authors were supported in part by a Grant from the Research and Educational Fund of the Department of Oral and Maxillofacial Surgery, Massachussets General Hospital, Boston, Massachussets. Partial support was received for the preparation of this article through a grant from "The Coverys Community Healthcare Foundation".

## REFERENCES

1. Keith DA, Shannon TA, Kulich R. The prescription monitoring program data: what it can tell you. J Am Dent Assoc 2018;149(4):266–72.
2. National Association of Boards of Pharmacy. Available at: https://nabp.pharmacy/wp-content/uploads/2019/04/PMP-InterConnect-Map-August-2019.pdf. Accessed December 30, 2019.
3. Mass.gov. Massachusetts prescription monitoring program. Available at: http://www.mass.gov/eohhs/gov/departments/dph/programs/hcq/drug-control/pmp/. Accessed December 18, 2019.
4. The Pew Charitable Trusts. States require opioid prescribers to check for 'doctor shopping.'. Available at: http://www.pewtrusts.org/en/research-and-analysis/blogs/stateline/2016/05/09/states-require-opioid-prescribersto-check-for-doctor-shopping. Accessed December 18, 2019.

5. U.S. Food & Drug Administration. FDA requires strong warnings for opioid analgesics, prescription opioid cough products, and benzodiazepine labeling related to serious risks and death from combined use: action to better inform prescribers and protect patients as part of agency's opioid action plan. Available at: https://www.fda.gov/NewsEvents/Newsroom/PressAnnouncements/ucm518697.htm. Accessed December 18, 2019.

6. U.S. Department of Health and Human Services, Centers for Disease Control and Prevention. CDC guideline for prescribing opioids for chronic pain. Available at: https://www.cdc.gov/drugoverdose/pdf/guidelines_at-a-glance-a.pdf. Accessed December 18, 2019.

7. Dunn KM, Saunders KW, Rutter CM, et al. Opioid prescriptions for chronic pain and overdose: a cohort study. Ann Intern Med 2010;152(2):85–92.

8. Mass.gov. Massachusetts prescription monitoring program. Visano. Available at: https://www.mass.gov/guides/massachusetts-prescription-awareness-tool-masspat#-visano—new-masspat-enhancement-. Accessed December 30, 2019.

9. Siegel R, Cheung J. Dental schools add an urgent lesson: think twice about prescribing opioids. Available at: http://www.npr.org/sections/health-shots/2017/09/08/549218604/dental-schools-add-an-urgent-lesson-thinktwice-about-prescribing-opioids. Accessed December 18, 2019.

10. Drugabuse.gov. Opioid risk tool. Available at: https://www.drugabuse.gov/sites/default/files/files/OpioidRiskTool.pdf. Accessed December 18, 2019.

11. Kulich RJ, Backstrom J, Brownstein J, et al. A model for opioid risk stratification: assessing the psychosocial components of orofacial pain. Oral Maxillofac Surg Clin North Am 2016;28(3):261–73.

12. National Institute on Drug Abuse. Resource guide: screening for drug use in general medical settings. The NIDA Quick Screen. Available at: https://www.drugabuse.gov/publications/resource-guide-screening-drug-use-ingeneral-medical-settings/nida-quick-screen. Accessed December 18, 2019.

13. Finley EP, Garcia A, Rosen K, et al. Evaluating the impact of prescription drug monitoring program implementation: a scoping review. BMC Health Serv Res 2017;17(1):420.

14. Rasubala L, Pernapati L, Velasquez X, et al. Impact of a mandatory prescription drug monitoring program on prescription of opioid analgesics by dentists. PLoS One 2015;10(8):e0135957.

15. Greenwood-Ericksen MB, Poon SJ, Nelson LS, et al. Best practices for prescription drug monitoring programs in the emergency department setting: results of an expert panel. Ann Emerg Med 2016;67(6):755–64.

16. Fink PB, Deyo RA, Hallvik SE, et al. Opioid prescribing patterns and patient outcomes by prescriber type in the Oregon prescription drug monitoring program. Pain Med 2018;19(12):2481–6.

17. Hawk K, D'onofrio G, Fiellin DA, et al. Past-year prescription drug monitoring program opioid prescriptions and self-reported opioid use in an emergency department population with opioid use disorder. Acad Emerg Med 2018;25(5):508–16.

18. Massachusetts Department of Public Health. The Massachusetts Substance Use Helpline. Available at: https://www.helplinema.org. Accessed December 31, 2019.

19. U.S. Department of Health and Human Services, Centers for Disease Control and Prevention. Opioid Overdose. Mobile App. Available at: https://www.cdc.gov/drugoverdose/prescribing/app.html. Accessed December 31, 2019.

20. McCauley JL, Leite RS, Melvin CL, et al. Dental opioid prescribing practices and risk mitigation strategy implementation: identification of potential targets for provider-level intervention. Subst Abus 2016;37(1):9–14.
21. Hoang E, Keith DA, Kulich R. Controlled substance misuse risk assessment and prescription monitoring database use by dentists. J Am Dent Assoc 2019;150(5): 383–92.
22. Prescription drug monitoring frequently asked questions (FAQ). Available at: http://www.pdmpassist.org. Accessed December 5, 2019.
23. Physicians' and pharmacists' liability National Alliance for Model State Drug Laws. Available at: http://www.namsdl.org/library/80E5C482-19B9-E1C5-3115CF5FF9E4AD22. Accessed December 5, 2019.
24. Keith DA, Kulich RJ, Bharel M, et al. Massachusetts dental schools respond to the prescription opioid crisis: a statewide collaboration. J Dental Educ 2017;81: 1388–94.

# Managing Acute Dental Pain

## Principles for Rational Prescribing and Alternatives to Opioid Therapy

Shehryar Nasir Khawaja, BDS, MSc[a],
Steven John Scrivani, DDS, DMSc[b,c],*

## KEYWORDS

- Dental pain • Opioid therapy • Analgesics • Non-Narcotic drug combinations

## KEY POINTS

- Pharmacotherapy forms an integral part of acute dental pain management.
- For an appropriate pain management regimen, it is essential to consider the underlying cause of pain, and the medical and medication history of the patient.
- Mostly safe and effective management of acute dental pain can be accomplished with a non-opioid medication regimen. However, in certain circumstances opioid-medication regimen is needed.
- Opioids result in strong analgesia. However, they have a significant adverse effect profile, and can interact and potentiate the depressant effects of other centrally-acting medications.
- Pain management regimens, such as pre-emptive analgesia, post-procedural cold-compression, long-acting anesthetic and compound drug therapy can improve the efficacy of analgesics without compromising patient safety.

## INTRODUCTION

Acute pain is inherent in dentistry. Definitive treatment consists primarily of surgical dental procedures. Analgesic medications, however, often form an intricate part of the treatment strategy.[1] Safe and effective management of acute pain can be accomplished using non–opioid-based and opioid-based analgesics.[2] To formulate a pharmacologic plan, a thorough history and physical examination, in addition to

[a] Orofacial Pain Medicine, Department of Internal Medicine, Shaukat Khanum Memorial Cancer Hospital and Research Centre, 7A Block R-3 M.A. Johar Town, Lahore, Punjab 54782, Pakistan; [b] Department of Diagnostic Sciences, Craniofacial Pain Center, Tufts University School of Dental Medicine, 1 Kneeland Street, Boston, MA 02111, USA; [c] Pain Research, Education and Policy Program, Department of Public Health and Community Medicine, Tufts University School of Medicine, Boston, MA, USA
* Corresponding author. Department of Diagnostic Sciences, Craniofacial Pain Center, Tufts University School of Dental Medicine, 1 Kneeland Street, Boston, MA 02111.
E-mail address: sjscrivani1@gmail.com

Dent Clin N Am 64 (2020) 525–534
https://doi.org/10.1016/j.cden.2020.02.003
0011-8532/20/© 2020 Elsevier Inc. All rights reserved.

appropriate investigations, are essential. This article reviews the pharmacology of non–opioid-based and opioid-based analgesics and the use of additional strategies to enhance therapeutic response required for optimal pain relief. These guidelines are in concordance with those published by American Dental Association.[2]

## EVALUATION OF ACUTE DENTAL PAIN

There is a broad differential diagnosis for dental, oral, and facial pain. Many of these conditions have unique and distinctive characteristics that typically distinguish them.[3,4] In order to diagnose the cause of dental pain accurately, careful and thorough history and examination are required. These should be supplemented with appropriate and valid clinical and radiological investigations.[5]

## MANAGEMENT OF ACUTE DENTAL CONDITIONS

Once diagnosis and cause of acute dental pain have been established, appropriate dental treatment should be undertaken. This usually results in rapid de-escalation of symptoms and resolution of the disease process. In addition, there may be need for pain control, prior to, during, or after definitive treatments.[1,6] The use of analgesic drugs to manage pain should be restricted to appropriate medications, dosage, and number of pills and used, whenever possible, as an adjunct to the definitive dental treatment. Most of the acute painful dental conditions that require analgesics are secondary to inflammation in the pulp, periodontal ligament space, or associated tissues. The inflammation can be a consequence of infection, trauma, or operative procedure. Contingent on the etiology of the underlying cause, pain medications may need to be used in conjunction with other medications, for example, the presence of infection may necessitate the use of antibiotics.

The medications used most frequently for management of acute dental pain consist of acetaminophen, nonsteroidal anti-inflammatory drugs (NSAIDs), opioids, and combination therapy (**Table 1**).

## ACETAMINOPHEN

Acetaminophen is a centrally acting analgesic. There is limited understanding, however, regarding the exact site and mechanism of its action. It has been postulated that it depresses nociceptive activity evoked in thalamic neurons by electrical stimulation of nociceptive afferents and also may result in central analgesia (independent of endogenous opioids). Likewise, it has been suggested that it inhibits the function of cyclooxygenase-3 enzymes. However, genomic and kinetic analyses indicate this inhibitory effect to be clinically irrelevant.[1,6,7]

Single doses of acetaminophen are effective analgesics for acute postoperative pain. The number needed to treat (NNT) after a single dose of acetaminophen, 500 mg, was 3.5 (2.7–4.8). For acute dental pain, acetaminophen, 975 mg to 1000 mg, the NNT was 3.6 (3.2–4.1). Multiple studies have suggested acetaminophen, 975 mg to 1000 mg, has a similar analgesic effect to aspirin, 650 mg. Conversely, other studies have found ibuprofen, 400 mg, and diclofenac, 50 mg, superior to acetaminophen in reducing pain and swelling in patients undergoing third molar extraction.[1,6,8]

Acetaminophen is a relatively safe medication, with a large therapeutic window and fewer long-term gastrointestinal side effects. Common adverse effects include rash and hypothermia. Long-term use of acetaminophen has been associated with renal and hepatic issues. Caution is advised in alcohol abusers (>3 alcoholic drinks per

**Table 1**
**The number needed to treat after a single dose of medication for treatment of acute dental pain**

| Medication | Number Needed to Treat (95% CI) |
|---|---|
| Acetaminophen, 1000 mg, with ibuprofen, 400 mg | 1.5 (1.4–1.7) |
| Acetaminophen, 1000 mg, with oxycodone, 10 mg | 1.8 (1.6–2.2) |
| Ibuprofen, 200 mg, with caffeine, 100 mg | 2.1 (1.8–2.5) |
| Ibuprofen, 400 mg, with oxycodone, 5 mg | 2.2 (1.8–2.9) |
| Acetaminophen, 1000 mg, with codeine, 60 mg | 2.2 (1.8–2.9) |
| Diclofenac, 50 mg | 2.3 (2.0–2.7) |
| Oxycodone, 15 mg | 2.4 (1.4–4.4) |
| Ibuprofen, 400 mg | 2.4 (2.3–2.6) |
| Naproxen, 550 mg | 2.6 (2.2–3.2) |
| Acetaminophen, 650–975 mg, with tramadol, 75 mg | 2.6 (2.3–3.0) |
| Acetaminophen, 500 mg | 3.5 (2.7–4.8) |
| Acetaminophen, 1000 mg | 3.6 (3.2–4.1) |
| Celecoxib, 200 mg | 4.2 (3.4–5.6) |
| Tramadol, 75 mg | 9.9 (6.9–17.0) |
| Codeine, 60 mg | 12.0 |
| Codeine, 30 mg | 16.7 |

day) and in patients with liver disease. Acetaminophen is the analgesic of choice during pregnancy or lactation (pregnancy category B). Recent studies suggest, however, that high-dose usage in the third trimester may result in premature ductus arteriosus closure.[1,6,8]

Acetaminophen is available in various combinations. Acetaminophen plus caffeine (20 mg–65 mg) has shown superior to acetaminophen alone in management of acute dental pain, but it was found similar to ibuprofen. Similarly, acetaminophen plus codeine (30 mg) has been shown superior to NSAIDs, acetaminophen alone, and acetaminophen with caffeine. The NNT of acetaminophen, 800 mg to 1000 mg, plus codeine, 60 mg, was 2.2 (1.8–2.9). The analgesic effectiveness of acetaminophen also has been studied in combination with NSAIDs, such as ibuprofen. Acetaminophen and ibuprofen combinations have been shown to have more analgesic efficacy than acetaminophen-codeine and ibuprofen-codeine combinations and than oxycodone alone. The NNT of acetaminophen, 1000 mg, and ibuprofen, 400 mg, was 1.5 (1.4–1.7).[8–10]

To summarize, acetaminophen alone, at 500-mg to 1000-mg oral dosage (every 4–6 hours, as needed to a maximum of 4000 mg/d), is appropriate for management of mild to moderate acute dental pain. Furthermore, in combination with other agents, such as caffeine, or analgesics, such as NSAIDs and opioids, it can be used for management of severe acute dental pain.

## NONSTEROIDAL ANTI-INFLAMMATORY DRUGS

NSAIDs are a group of analgesics that function by inhibiting enzymatic activity of cyclooxygenase (COX)-1 and COX-2 enzymes. COX enzymes are responsible for production of prostaglandins, which are associated with pain and inflammation. NSAIDs either can specifically block a particular type of enzyme (COX-2 selective NSAIDs) or have a generalized inhibitory effect on both COX-1 and COX-2 enzymes (nonselective NSAIDs).[11,12]

Commonly used NSAIDs include ibuprofen, naproxen, diclofenac, and celecoxib. Ibuprofen, naproxen, and diclofenac are nonselective COX inhibitors. Ibuprofen is an effective analgesic and available in various strengths. The NNT for ibuprofen, 400 mg, in managing acute dental pain has been established to be 2.4 (2.3–2.6). This has shown superior to acetaminophen, 1000 mg, and aspirin, 600 mg to 650 mg. Naproxen has analgesic efficacy and onset similar to ibuprofen. The NNT of naproxen, 550 mg, for management of acute pain was found to be 2.6 (2.2–3.2). Diclofenac, as discussed previously, is a nonselective NSAID; however, it has a preferential inhibitory nature toward COX-2 enzymes. Nonetheless, the efficacy of diclofenac is similar to that of ibuprofen and naproxen. The NNT of diclofenac, 50 mg, was calculated to be 2.3 (2.0–2.7) for managing acute dental pain. Currently, the only COX-2 selective NSAID available is celecoxib. It has been shown effective in controlling postprocedure pain and inflammation. The effectiveness of celecoxib, however, in comparison to conventional nonselective NSAIDs has been inferior. The NNT for celecoxib, 200 mg, has been reported to be 4.2 (3.4–5.6).[8]

NSAIDs can be associated with multiple adverse effects. This is due to the interference of NSAIDs with the production of prostaglandins and thromboxanes. Furthermore, they result in upregulation of leukotrienes, which are responsible for inducing hyperalgesia and sensitivity reactions. Recent studies have suggested, however, that the occurrence of such adverse effects is low. There were no statistically significant differences observed in occurrence of adverse effects between ibuprofen, 400 mg; naproxen, 500 mg to 550 mg; diclofenac, 25 mg to 75 mg; and placebo. Common side effects associated with nonselective NSAIDs are due to inhibition of prostaglandins including gastrointestinal toxicity (diarrhea, constipation, abdominal pain, ulceration, heartburn, nausea, and vomiting) and renal failure. Inhibition of thromboxanes may result in prolonged bleeding and increase in leukotriene levels can result in hypersensitivity reactions, such as asthma and utricaria. Other common side effects associated with use of NSAIDs include, rash, tinnitus, somnolence, and dizziness. COX-2 selective NSAIDs have relatively less acute gastrointestinal side effects. They are associated, however, with increase in cardiovascular events, such as myocardial infarction and ischemic stroke. Relative contraindications for use of NSAIDs include a history of asthma, renal disease, gastrointestinal bleeding, ulceration or perforation, and cardiovascular disease. Use of NSAIDs should be avoided during pregnancy. They have been reported to increase risk for perinatal mortality, neonatal hemorrhage, decreased birth weight, prolonged gestation and labor, and possible teratogenicity.[11–13]

NSAIDs have been studied as combination analgesics. Studies have suggested that analgesic effectiveness of ibuprofen is enhanced with the addition of acetaminophen, caffeine, and opioid-based analgesics. The NNTs for these combinations were calculated to be 1.5 (1.4–1.7), 2.1 (1.8–2.5), and 2.2 (1.8–2.9), respectively.[8,14,15]

To summarize, commonly used NSAIDs are appropriate for management of moderate-severe intensity, acute dental pain. They are associated with various adverse effects; however, the prevalence of such events has been reported to be low. For patients with severe acute pain, NSAIDs can be used in combination with other agents, such as caffeine, acetaminophen, and opioids.

## OPIOID ANALGESICS

Opioids are a group of medications that produce analgesia by acting on the opioid receptors. There are 3 major classes of opioid receptors: mu, kappa, and delta. These are distributed across several levels of the nervous system and in many peripheral tissues. Opioids inhibit release of neurotransmitters from the primary afferent nerve terminals and activate the descending inhibitory controls in the midbrain. A majority of opioid medications exert their analgesic response by binding preferentially to the mu receptors. Morphine has the highest relative preference for the mu receptors. Codeine has a poor binding capability to mu receptors, however, and for this reason it is considered a prodrug, which eventually metabolizes into morphine to exert its pharmacologic action. Likewise, oxycodone metabolizes into oxymorphone and exerts its antinociceptive response via kappa receptors. Tramadol, unlike the rest of the opioids, is a synthetic centrally acting opioid analgesic. It binds poorly to mu receptors and has low affinity for delta and kappa receptors. It induces its analgesic response by additionally inhibiting norepinephrine and serotonin pathways in the central nervous system.[16]

Several investigations have been conducted on the effectiveness of opioids on the management of acute dental pain. Examples of commonly used opioids include codeine, oxycodone, hydrocodone, and tramadol. Codeine has been studied alone and in combinations with acetaminophen and NSAIDs. Recommended dose for codeine is 30 mg to 60 mg, every 4 hours to 8 hours. It has poor analgesic effectiveness, however, when used alone for management of acute dental pain. The NNTs for codeine, 30 mg and 60 mg, alone to relieve acute dental pain have been established to be 16.7 and 12, respectively. As a combination analgesic with acetaminophen, 1000 mg, plus codeine, 60 mg, however, it was found significantly better, with an NNT of 2.2 (1.8–2.9). Likewise, tramadol, 75 mg to 112.5 mg, has shown to have a poor antinociceptive effect on the management of moderate to severe acute dental postoperative pain. The NNT for tramadol, 75 mg, to relieve acute dental pain by 50% was calculated to be 9.9 (6.9–17). This improved significantly with combination with acetaminophen, 650 mg to 975 mg. The NNT for this combination was 2.6 (2.3–3). It was statistically similar, however, in efficacy to the analgesic effect of ibuprofen, 400 mg.[1,6,8]

Oxycodone is considered a relatively strong opioid. The recommended dose is 5 mg to 15 mg every 4 hours to 8 hours. Oxycodone, 5 mg, however, has been shown to not have any beneficial effect in management of acute postoperative pain. On the other hand, a single dose of oxycodone, 15 mg, may provide significant relief in symptoms. The NNT for oxycodone, 15 mg, to result in at least 50% relief in symptoms in patients with moderate to severe postoperative pain was reported to be 2.4 (1.4–4.4). This was similar to the NNT for oxycodone, 10 mg, with acetaminophen, 650 mg, combination therapy. Hydrocodone is another strong opioid that commonly is used in combination in the management of acute dental pain. The recommended dose for hydrocodone is 7.5 mg to 15 mg every 4 hours to 8 hours. Hydrocodone, 7.5 mg, with acetaminophen, 500 mg, has been shown superior to placebo in managing moderate to severe postoperative pain. It was found inferior, however, to the efficacy of oxycodone, 5 mg, plus ibuprofen, 400 mg, and ketorolac, 10 mg.[1,6,8,15]

The use of the opioids is associated with several adverse effects. These are dose-dependent effects, so the incidence varies. The severity and inconvenience of these effects often are high. Studies on opioids have reported up to 22% patients withdrawing due to intolerance to opioids induced adverse effects. Furthermore, studies comparing acetaminophen, NSAIDs, and opioids reported that most adverse effects took place in patients using opioids. Short-term opioid use commonly is associated with gastrointestinal issues (nausea, vomiting, constipation, and dry mouth), respiratory depression, somnolence, headache, itching, and mood changes (dysphoria and euphoria). Long-term opioid use has been associated with physical dependence and tolerance, hormonal imbalance, and potential drug abuse. The relative contraindications for using the opioids are severe chronic respiratory disease, severe inflammatory bowel disease, and concurrent use of alcohol and cannabis.[8]

Opioid analgesics may interact with other medications through multiple mechanisms. These can take place from induction or inhibition of the hepatic cytochrome P450 monooxygenase system. Opioids undergo hepatic metabolism, and drug interactions affecting this mechanism can have a clinically significant effect. For example, antibiotics, such as erythromycin, can increase the effect of opioids, and rifampicin, carbamazepine, and barbiturates can decrease the effect of opioids. Likewise, concurrent use of centrally acting medications, such as benzodiazepine, tricyclic antidepressants, serotonin and norepinephrine uptake inhibitors, hypnotics, muscle relaxants, and monoamine oxidase inhibitors, increases the risk of profound central nervous system and respiratory depression, psychomotor impairment, and severe constipation and alters seizure control.[17]

Irrespective of the duration of use, opioid use is associated with potential for accidental overdose and death. Given the relative ratio of therapeutic benefits versus risks, the opioids are not considered the analgesic of choice in management of acute dental pain. They should be used as an adjunct to nonopioid medications, such as acetaminophen and NSAIDs, and their use should be limited to second line or third line of therapy in management of severe acute dental pain. Several opioid-based combinations have been studied for management of acute dental pain. Most effective combinations are acetaminophen, 1000 mg, plus oxycodone, 10 mg (NNT of 1.8 [1.6–2.2]); acetaminophen, 1000 mg, plus codeine, 60 mg (NNT of 2.2 [1.8–2.9]); ibuprofen, 400 mg, plus codeine, 60 mg (NNT of 2.2 [1.8–2.6]); and ibuprofen, 400 mg, plus oxycodone, 10 mg (NNT of 2.3 [2–2.8]).[8] Caution is advised, however, when using opioid-based combinations, because they have been associated with significantly more adverse effects than placebo controls. This is contrary to non–opioid-based combinations that have shown to have significantly fewer such effects than placebo.

## COMBINATION DRUG THERAPY

As discussed previously, several combinations of analgesics (opioid-based and non–opioid-based) have been investigated in the management of acute dental pain. Studies have suggested that combination drug therapy improves analgesic efficacy, facilitates better absorption of medications, decreases likelihood of adverse effects, reduces cost of care, allows concurrent management of multiple symptoms, and improves patient adherence to the recommended pharmacologic plan.[2,10]

There are multiple mechanisms that allow combination drug therapy to be superior to single-agent analgesic therapy. There is additive effect when 2 pharmacologically different analgesic agents are used in combination. The pain pathway is complex, with multiple pathways that are activated or inhibited from the point nociceptive signals are generated to the point where pain is processed and interpreted in the prefrontal cortex.[18] Specific analgesics act on particular set of receptors that are spread across these pathways. By using 2 different pharmacologic analgesics, more than 1 type of pathway is targeted. This clinically translates as improved and more extensive analgesia than either agent used alone. Similarly, it has been postulated that when analgesics are used in combination, 1 drug alters the nociceptive sensitivity of the other medication. For example, NSAIDs alter the form of COX enzymes. This alteration provides greater sensitivity to acetaminophen, resulting in a synergistic analgesic response.

Lastly, pharmacogenetics plays a role in success of combination drug therapy. Genetic variations in sensitivity or metabolism of medications play a vital role in a patient experiencing better response to 1 medication or another. Genetic polymorphisms may result in a patient not having the specific enzymes required for metabolic activation of a prodrug. For example, approximately 8% to 10% of the population does not have enzymes required for metabolism of codeine to morphine. In combination analgesic therapy, however, there is a likelihood that at least 1 of the agents will result in pain relief.[10]

One of the most effective and safest combinations in terms of incidence of adverse effects is the combination of acetaminophen plus ibuprofen. Acetaminophen, 1000 mg, with ibuprofen, 400 mg, has shown superior to ibuprofen, 400 mg, plus codeine, 25.6 mg; acetaminophen, 1000 mg, plus codeine, 30 mg; and acetaminophen or ibuprofen alone in providing relief in acute dental pain. In addition, a recent systematic review has suggested that acetaminophen plus ibuprofen, in both 1000 mg and 400 mg, respectively, and 500 mg and 200 mg, respectively, strengths, have the least NNTs, 1.5 (1.4–1.7) and 1.6 (1.5–1.8), respectively.[8,10] This review reported that both these combinations had statistically less incidence of adverse effects than placebo controls.[8] Due to this, it is recommended as first-line pharmacotherapy for management of moderate or severe acute dental pain.

## ROLE OF PREEMPTIVE ANALGESIA

Preemptive analgesia is defined as a treatment modality that is initiated before a traumatic event, such as surgical incision or extraction, is introduced. The intention is to preempt the establishment of peripheral and central sensitization while leaving physiologic nociceptive mechanisms intact so that they can continue to function as an early warning system.[17] Studies on preemptive analgesia suggest that it results in more extensive analgesia during the procedure, delays the time to first analgesic after intervention, reduces postprocedural consumption of analgesics, improves postsurgical swelling, and lessens medication-associated adverse effects. Multiple medications have been investigated as preemptive analgesics. Current literature suggests that acetaminophen, NSAIDs, gabapentinoids, opioids, and corticosteroids can be used as preemptive analgesics.[13,19–21]

Preemptive analgesics are administered 1 hour to 3 hours before the time of procedure. The recommended dosages for preemptive analgesics are provided in **Table 2**.

## OTHER ANALGESIC MODALITIES TO AID IN PAIN CONTROL

Recently, long-acting anesthetic (lasting for approximately 72 hours post–administration of injection) has been shown helpful in management of acute postsurgical pain associated with third molar extraction.[22] Liposomal bupivacaine is a prolonged-release formulation of bupivacaine. It has been shown helpful in management of acute postsurgical pain associated with bilateral third molar extraction. The anesthetic is intended for use as an infiltration into the surgical site. It is available as a 13.3-mg/mL solution in either a 20-mL or 10-mL vial. The anesthetic solution consists of a combination of intraliposomal bupivacaine (97%) and extraliposomal bupivacaine (3%). The intraliposomal bupivacaine is entrapped inside vesicles and surrounded by a lipid bilayer. Once injected, these liposomes undergo gradual breakdown and release slowly in the injected tissue. Meanwhile, free extraliposomal bupivacaine interacts with sensory receptors immediately post–administration of anesthetic. Due to this, the anesthetic has a bimodal plasma concentration–versus–time curve, with 1 peak at approximately 1 hour after administration and a second peak at approximately 12 hours to 36 hours. The concentration of bupivacaine

**Table 2**
Doses of medications that can be used as preemptive analgesics for management of acute dental pain

| Medication | Dose (mg) |
|---|---|
| Acetaminophen | 1000 |
| Ibuprofen | 400–600 |
| Diclofenac | 50–75 |
| Dexamethasone | 2–8 |
| Pregabalin | 75–150 |
| Gabapentin | 600–900 |
| Tramadol | 75–100 |

decreases slowly and is detectable for up to 72 hours to 96 hours, depending on the site of administration.[23,24]

Postprocedural cryotherapy in the form of ice compressions or hilotherapy may help in reducing postoperative swelling and pain associated with intraoral surgery.[25–27] The therapeutic effect is attributed to alteration in hemodynamic, neuromuscular, and metabolic processes. Furthermore, studies have suggested that cold temperature decreases the excitability of free nerve endings and peripheral nerve fibers.[28]

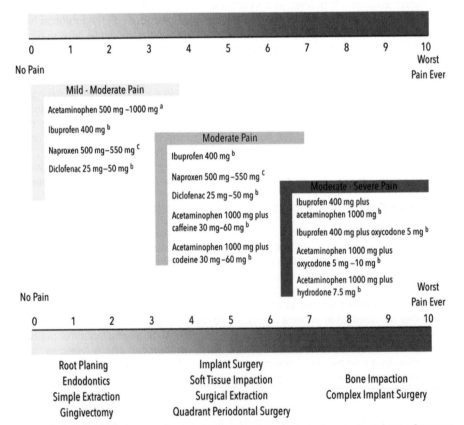

**Fig. 1.** Recommended pharmacologic strategy for management of acute dental pain. [a] Repeat every 4–6 hours. [b] Repeat every 8 hours. [c] Repeat every 12 hours.

## SUMMARY

Treatment of acute dental pain consists primarily of definitive dental (surgical) therapy. In many situations, however, the use of analgesic medications forms an intricate part of the treatment strategy. Safe and effective management of acute pain can be accomplished using pharmacologic (non–opioid-based and opioid-based analgesics and long-acting anesthetics) and nonpharmacologic (ice compressions and hilotherapy) modalities. For mild to moderate pain, a rational choice is acetaminophen, 500 mg to 1000 mg, every 4 to 6 hours. Alternatives are provided in **Fig. 1**. For moderate to severe pain, ideal choice are NSAIDs, such as, ibuprofen, 400 mg, every 8 hours; naproxen, 500 mg to 550 mg, every 12 hours; and diclofenac, 25 mg to 50 mg, every 8 to 12 hours. For severe pain, the first choice is a combination analgesic, such as acetaminophen, 1000 mg, plus ibuprofen, 400 mg, every 8 hours. Other non–opioid-based and opioid-based combinations can be used as well. Furthermore, if acute dental pain is expected after a procedure, dentists always should consider use of preemptive analgesics, postsurgical long-acting anesthesia, and ice compression. For additional information please refer to the American Dental Association manual on safe prescribing and substance use disorders.

## FUNDING

Partial support was received for the preparation of this article through a grant from "The Coverys Community Healthcare Foundation."

## DISCLOSURE

The authors have nothing to disclose.

## REFERENCES

1. Hargreaves K, Abbott PV. Drugs for pain management in dentistry. Aust Dent J 2005;50(4 Suppl 2):S14–22.

2. O'Neil M, American Dental Association, editors. The ADA practical guide to substance use disorders and safe prescribing. Hoboken (NJ): John Wiley and Sons Inc; 2015.

3. Tal M, Devor M. Chapter 2 - Anatomy and neurophysiology of orofacial pain A2 - Sharav, Yair. In: Benoliel R, editor. Orofacial pain and headache. Edinburgh (Scotland): Mosby; 2008. p. 19–44.

4. Sharav Y, Benoliel R. Chapter 5 - Acute orofacial pain. In: Sharav Y, Benoliel R, editors. Orofacial pain and headache. Edinburgh (Scotland): Mosby; 2008. p. 75–90.

5. Idahosa CN, Kerr AR. Clinical evaluation of oral diseases. In: Farah CS, Balasubramaniam R, McCullough MJ, editors. Contemporary oral medicine. Cham (Switzerland): Springer International Publishing; 2019. p. 137–71.

6. Haas DA. An update on analgesics for the management of acute postoperative dental pain. J Can Dent Assoc 2002;68(8):476–82.

7. Botting RM. Mechanism of action of acetaminophen: is there a cyclooxygenase 3? Clin Infect Dis 2000;31(Supplement 5):S202–10.

8. Moore PA, Ziegler KM, Lipman RD, et al. Benefits and harms associated with analgesic medications used in the management of acute dental pain: An overview of systematic reviews. J Am Dent Assoc 2018;149(4):256–65.e3.

9. Ong CK, Seymour RA, Lirk P, et al. Combining paracetamol (acetaminophen) with nonsteroidal antiinflammatory drugs: a qualitative systematic review of analgesic efficacy for acute postoperative pain. Anesth Analg 2010;110(4):1170–9.

10. Moore PA, Hersh EV. Combining ibuprofen and acetaminophen for acute pain management after third-molar extractions: translating clinical research to dental practice. J Am Dent Assoc 2013;144(8):898–908.

11. Kallings P. Nonsteroidal anti-inflammatory drugs. Vet Clin North Am Equine Pract 1993;9(3):523–41.

12. Naesdal J, Brown K. NSAID-associated adverse effects and acid control aids to prevent them: a review of current treatment options. Drug Saf 2006;29(2):119–32.

13. Dahl JB, Nielsen RV, Wetterslev J, et al. Post-operative analgesic effects of paracetamol, NSAIDs, glucocorticoids, gabapentinoids and their combinations: a topical review. Acta Anaesthesiol Scand 2014;58(10):1165–81.

14. Derry S, Wiffen PJ, Moore RA. Single dose oral ibuprofen plus caffeine for acute postoperative pain in adults. Cochrane Database of Systematic Reviews. 2015

15. Litkowski LJ, Christensen SE, Adamson DN, et al. Analgesic efficacy and tolerability of oxycodone 5 mg/ibuprofen 400 mg compared with those of oxycodone 5 mg/acetaminophen 325 mg and hydrocodone 7.5 mg/acetaminophen 500 mg in patients with moderate to severe postoperative pain: a randomized, double-blind, placebo-controlled, single-dose, parallel-group study in a dental pain model. Clin Ther 2005;27(4):418–29.

16. Trescot AM, Datta S, Lee M, et al. Opioid pharmacology. Pain Physician 2008; 11(2 Suppl):S133–53.

17. Maurer PM, Bartkowski RR. Drug interactions of clinical significance with opioid analgesics. Drug Saf 1993;8(1):30–48.

18. Lorenz J, Minoshima S, Casey K. Keeping pain out of mind: the role of the dorsolateral prefrontal cortex in pain modulation. Brain 2003;126(5):1079–91.

19. Woolf CJ, Chong MS. Preemptive analgesia–treating postoperative pain by preventing the establishment of central sensitization. Anesth Analg 1993;77(2):362–79.

20. Kehlet H, Jensen TS, Woolf CJ. Persistent postsurgical pain: risk factors and prevention. Lancet 2006;367(9522):1618–25.

21. Ong CK, Lirk P, Seymour RA, et al. The efficacy of preemptive analgesia for acute postoperative pain management: a meta-analysis. Anesth Analg 2005;100(3): 757–73.

22. Lieblich SE, Danesi H. Liposomal bupivacaine use in third molar impaction surgery: INNOVATE study. Anesth Prog 2017;64(3):127–35.

23. Hu D, Onel E, Singla N, et al. Pharmacokinetic profile of liposome bupivacaine injection following a single administration at the surgical site. Clin Drug Investig 2013;33(2):109–15.

24. Chahar P, Cummings KC III. Liposomal bupivacaine: a review of a new bupivacaine formulation. J Pain Res 2012;5:257.

25. Forouzanfar T, Sabelis A, Ausems S, et al. Effect of ice compression on pain after mandibular third molar surgery: a single-blind, randomized controlled trial. Int J Oral Maxillofac Surg 2008;37(9):824–30.

26. Glass GE, Waterhouse N, Shakib K. Hilotherapy for the management of perioperative pain and swelling in facial surgery: a systematic review and meta-analysis. Br J Oral Maxillofac Surg 2016;54(8):851–6.

27. Greenstein G. Therapeutic efficacy of cold therapy after intraoral surgical procedures: a literature review. J Periodontol 2007;78(5):790–800.

28. Lee JM, Warren MP, Mason SM. Effects of ice on nerve conduction velocity. Physiotherapy 1978;64(1):2–6.

# Comorbid Conditions in Relation to Controlled Substance Abuse

Matthew Fortino, MA[a,b,c,*], Ronald J. Kulich, PhD[a,b,c],
Joshua A. Kaufman, MD[d], Hudson Franca, MD[e,f]

## KEYWORDS

- Brief intervention • Overdose • Prescreen • Referral • SBIRT • Screening
- Substance use disorder

## KEY POINTS

- Comorbid medical disease and psychiatric disorders are associated with an elevated likelihood of a patient's misuse and abuse of controlled substances.
- Objective predictors can be assessed to inform dental practice and reduce the likelihood of overdose and the development/exacerbation of a substance use disorder.
- Dentists are advised to investigate substance use history with patients and manage the risk factors presented per a Controlled Substance Risk Mitigation checklist.

Psychiatric disorders can occur with the patient who also presents with simultaneous medical conditions, such as infections, gastrointestinal disorders, and other medical conditions. Both psychological and medical comorbidities can influence a patient's treatment adherence, perception of pain, postsurgery recovery, health care utilization, and mortality.[1,2] When more severe mental health and medical comorbidities are present, health care costs and utilization are increased, and eventually a "morbidity burden" for the patient is seen.[3]

A patient's biological, psychological, and social factors (biopsychosocial factors) impact the risk of developing a substance use disorder (SUD), along with the risk of

[a] Department of Oral and Maxillofacial Surgery, Tufts University School of Dental Medicine, 1 Kneeland Street, Boston, MA 02111, USA; [b] Department of Diagnostic Sciences, Tufts University School of Dental Medicine, Boston, MA, USA; [c] Department of Anesthesia, Critical Care and Pain Medicine, Harvard Medical School, Massachusetts General Hospital, 55 Fruit Street, 3rd Fl, Boston, MA 02114, USA; [d] Department of Psychiatry, Columbia University, New York State Psychiatric Institute, 1051 Riverside Dr, New York, New York 10032, USA; [e] Tufts University School of Dental Medicine, 1 Kneeland Street, Boston, MA 02111, USA; [f] Universidad Iberoamericana, Santo Domingo, Dominican Republic
* Corresponding author. Department of Oral and Maxillofacial Surgery, Tufts University School of Dental Medicine, 1 Kneeland Street, Boston, MA 02111.
*E-mail address:* mfortino@mgh.harvard.edu

Dent Clin N Am 64 (2020) 535–546
https://doi.org/10.1016/j.cden.2020.03.001
0011-8532/20/© 2020 Elsevier Inc. All rights reserved.

dental.theclinics.com

developing dental pathologic condition, for example, chronic masticatory dysfunction and temporomandibular disorders (TMD).[4] Within chronic pain populations, premorbid psychological factors, including depressed mood, perceived stress, and above all else, somatization, reliably predict the new-onset and persistence of TMD conditions to the degree that the relationship between TMD and psychological factors substantiate the claim of causality.[5] Patients with psychiatric diagnoses also pose a higher risk of presenting with decayed, missing, or filled teeth. For example, a sample of 5,076 patients with psychiatric diagnoses had a 2.8 greater likelihood of having lost all their teeth compared with the 39,545 persons in comparison groups.[6] These untoward consequences underscore the need for the dentist to better assess and manage a patient's psychiatric and medical comorbidities. The presence of these risk factors needs not derail treatment. Patients can be counseled when they are identified, with guidance on management in order to achieve better clinical outcome with overall dental care. In addition, communication with other health care providers should always occur, including the patient's primary treating medical clinicians or cotreating mental health practitioners.

When assessing risk for the development of SUD, dental practitioners typically tend to focus on the negative predictors that might be present. Conversely, some argue that more attention should be paid to positive factors that lower risk and promote successful treatment of a SUD. Similar to risk factors, protective factors are dynamic and longstanding conditions. Stability in family, interpersonal, and professional relationships are commonly recognized protective factors. Protective factors reduce the likelihood that an individual will abuse drugs. These elements need to be recognized by the clinician and reinforced with the patient.[7] Nonetheless, recognizing and reinforcing protective factors does not absolve the clinician of conducting a thorough assessment of controlled substance risks.

## SUBSTANCE USE DISORDER AND RELATED COMORBIDITIES

Most patients with severe mental illness may also display symptoms that meet the *Diagnostic and Statistical Manual of Mental Disorders* (Fifth Edition) criteria for SUD (**Box 1**).[8] Any mental disorder is considered serious when it imparts significant functional impairment that limits normative life activities. The authors typically see these impairments with psychotic disorders, schizophrenia, and moderate to severe depression.[9] SUDs are characterized by a pervasive display of behavioral and cognitive patterns, amid physiologic symptoms, that persist despite negative consequences of repeated drug use.[8] There are also specific, SUD-related criteria related to the effects of the particular substance being misused, for example, there is a difference between the intoxication and withdrawal properties of opioids versus alcohol.

As of 2019, nearly 20.3 million Americans aged 12 and older met criteria for an SUD. This number equates to ~8% of all Americans.[9] With drug initiation rates exceeding the birth rate, it is likely that dental practitioners will encounter patients who fall under this population statistic regardless of where they practice in the United States. The mortality from opioid overdose is shown to be even higher when the patient has other comorbid psychiatric disorders, including posttraumatic stress disorder (PTSD), bipolar disorder, and schizophrenia.[10]

It is estimated that more than 50% of psychiatric patients have a co-occuring SUD.[11] If the patient has 1 SUD, odds are that the patient also has a second.[11] For example, a patient who arrives at a dental practice with a history of longstanding alcohol use disorder may also be at greater risk for developing concomitant opioid use disorder. Among those with any lifetime SUD, 40% also had an anxiety disorder,

**Box 1**
**DSM-5 Diagnostic Criteria, Substance Use Disorder**

Other (or Unknown) Substance Use disorder

A. A problematic pattern of use of an intoxicating substance not able to be classified within the alcohol; caffeine; cannabis; hallucinogen (phencyclidine and others); inhalant; opioid; sedative, hypnotic, or anxiolytic; stimulant; or tobacco categories and leading to clinically significant impairment or distress, as manifested by at least two of the following, occurring within a 12-month period:

1. The substance is often taken in larger amounts or over a longer period than was intended.
2. There is a persistent desire or unsuccessful efforts to cut down or control use of the substance.
3. A great deal of time is spent in activities necessary to obtain the substance, use the substance, or recover from its effects.
4. Craving, or a strong desire or urge to use the substance.
5. Recurrent use of the substance resulting in a failure to fulfill major role obligations at work, school, or home.
6. Continued use of the substance despite having persistent or recurrent social or interpersonal problems caused or exacerbated by the effects of its use.
7. Important social, occupational, or recreational activities are given up or reduced because of use of the substance.
8. Recurrent use of the substance in situations in which it is physically hazardous.
9. Use of the substance is continued despite knowledge of having a persistent or recurrent physical or psychological problem that is likely to have been caused or exacerbated by the substance.
10. Tolerance, as defined by either of the following:
    a. A need for markedly increased amounts of the substance to achieve intoxication or desired effect.
    b. A markedly diminished effect with continued use of the same amount of the substance.
11. Withdrawal, as manifested by either of the following:
    a. The characteristic withdrawal syndrome for other (or unknown) substance (refer to Criteria A and B of the criteria sets for other [or unknown] substance withdrawal, p. 583).
    b. The substance (or a closely related substance) is taken to relieve or avoid withdrawal symptoms.

Specify if:
a) In early remission: After full criteria for other (or unknown) substance use disorder were previously met, none of the criteria for other (or unknown) substance use disorder have been met for at least 3 months but for less than 12 months (with the exception that Criterion A4, "Craving, or a strong desire or urge to use the substance," may be met).
b) In sustained remission: After full criteria for other (or unknown) substance use disorder were previously met, none of the criteria for other (or unknown) substance use disorder have been met at any time during a period of 12 months or longer (with the exception that Criterion A4, "Craving, or a strong desire or urge to use the substance," may be met).

Specify current severity/remission:
305.90 (F19.10) Mild: Presence of 2–3 symptoms.
(F19.11) Mild, In early remission
(F19.11) Mild, In sustained remission
304.90 (F19.20) Moderate: Presence of 4–5 symptoms.
(F19.21) Moderate, In early remission
(F19.21) Moderate, In sustained remission
304.90 (F19.20) Severe: Presence of 6 or more symptoms.
(F19.21) Severe, In early remission
(F19.21) Severe, In sustained remission

(Reprinted with permission from the Diagnostic and Statistical Manual of Mental Disorders, Fifth Edition, (Copyright ©2013). American Psychiatric Association. All Rights Reserved.)

and nearly 30% were found to have a mood disorder.[12] The odds of someone with a mood disorder having an SUD are 2.5 times greater than the general population.

Although opioids remain a major national concern, other legal and illicit drugs also deserve attention with regard to their risk for abuse and fatal overdose. More significantly, *polypharmacy* presents an increasing problem encountered in dental practice.[13] It typically manifests when a physician or dentist prescribes medications that may interact or complicate the patient risk status, for example, the combination of high-dose opioids and benzodiazepines results in an 8.9-fold increase in overdose risk.[14] Complicating the risk, each of the patient's health care providers may be unaware of medications not prescribed directly by them.

There are also cases whereby a single physician may be prescribing a complex regimen that increases patient risk. The authors have seen as many as 18 different controlled substances written by a single physician, occasionally with an added mix of different short and long-acting opioids. The overall dose exceeded the 90 morphine dose equivalent, a quantity suggestive of high overdose risk. The Centers for Disease Control and Prevention Guideline for Prescribing Opioids for Chronic Pain—United States, 2016, can offer guidance, specifically with respect to opioid dosing and polypharmacy, although there are controversies with respect to how effective the guideline has been implemented.[15] In the case noted above, the general dentist typically is not the clinician prescribing the high-dose opioids or prescribing concurrent multiple controlled substances. Nevertheless, the dentist should aware of the risk in order to provide better management of the patient and engage in effective communication with other cotreating providers.

## OTHER COMMON PSYCHIATRIC COMORBID DISORDERS

About 27% of dental patients report at least 1 mental illness, with anxiety reported second only to hypertension when considering all disease presentations. Following anxiety, commonly reported psychiatric disorders include depression, SUD's, PTSD, eating disorders, insomnia, and bipolar disorder. Somatic symptom disorders also are seen in dental practices, especially when treating persistent orofacial pain disorders. Characteristics can include the presence of marked somatic complaints, including multiple concurrent pain conditions in the context of conflicting medical and dental diagnoses. Patients may show anxiety and significant frustration, often as a result of visiting multiple health care providers. Again, a consequence may be polypharmacy and escalation of the patient's controlled substances by treating providers, the result being poor treatment outcome and increasing risk of an SUD.

### Anxiety and Depression

With 33.7% of the population experiencing an anxiety disorder in their life and an estimated 20% of adults diagnosed with an anxiety disorder in the past year,[16,17] a dentist can expect to encounter at least 1 patient with significant anxiety symptoms on a daily basis. In practice, anxiety persists as the most frequent comorbidity with only one-fourth of cases treated. Although dental practitioners tend to overfocus on dental phobias, other related anxiety disorders commonly cooccur with severe dental anxiety. The estimated 12-month prevalence of anxiety disorders in the general population ranges from about 11% to 18%, with a 1.5 to 2 times higher representation in women.[16,18] Distinguishable characteristics of an anxious patient typically take form through a protracted and amplified sympathetic arousal response, which develops into a fixed state of apprehension. The patient may report muscle tightness, elevated pain, fear, and avoidance of activity, as well as clusters of somatic complaints.

| Table 1 | | |
| --- | --- | --- |
| **Brief screening instruments** | | |
| **Screening Instruments** | **Definition** | **Time to Administer, min** |
| GAD-7 | 7-item instrument to assess generalized anxiety | 1–2 |
| PHQ-9 | 9-item instrument to measure depression symptoms | 1–2 |
| PHQ-2 | 2-item instrument to screen depressive symptoms | >1 |
| NIDA Quick Screen National Institute on Drug Abuse Quick Screen | 3-item instrument to measure drug use history and risk for SUD | 1–2 |
| SPRINT Short PTSD Rating Interview | 8-item instrument to measure core symptoms of PTSD, including somatic malaise, stress vulnerability, functional impairment | 1–2 |

*Data from* Refs.[45–48]

Although some level of apprehension is normal with dental procedures, a high level of severity may suggest the presence of a psychiatric disorder. The steps to identify severe anxiety include a combination of efficient history documentation and observation. The dentist may also easily identify the patient with a severe anxiety disorder when they arrive on multiple medications intended to target their symptoms. Brief anxiety screeners are available and easily adapted to dental practice. For example, the General Anxiety Disorder Scale, 7-Item (GAD-7) is commonly used in primary care medicine and can be easily administered by the dental hygienist or dentist (**Table 1**).

Following anxiety, depression is the second most frequent mental health disorder encountered by dentists. This finding comes as no surprise given the estimated 8% annual occurrence in the general population and 13.8% occurrence for young adults.[19] Major depressive disorder is defined as a period of severe and persistent low mood or anhedonia that persists daily for a period of 2 weeks. The symptoms cause impairment in social and occupational performance because of diminished social or occupational functioning capacity, which renders the sufferer with fatigue, the inability to experience pleasure, hopelessness, and sometimes suicidal ideation. Fluctuations in weight, irritability, and insomnia are common along with a reduced ability to concentrate. The patient may self-medicate with controlled substances in an effort to relieve their distress, and risk of SUD relapse is increased in the presence of a severe depressive episode. Depression and anxiety also commonly cooccur. Those with combined anxiety and depression may experience more severe symptoms, poorer social functioning, and lower remission rates than those who experience either disorder alone. If successful treatment of 1 disorder is carried out, then risk for developing a second one diminishes.[9]

A comorbid active SUD predicts poor treatment outcome for both anxiety and mood disorders. There is a well-established association between alcohol use disorder and a worsening major depressive disorder, although less than 1% of depressive disorders were found to be directly alcohol induced.[20] Both conditions are independent illnesses, and the clinician cannot assume that efforts to address active SUD would necessarily result in improvement of the patient's depression. Nonetheless, early recognition and management of depression can reduce risk of relapse with SUDs.

As with anxiety, there are brief screeners easily adapted to the dental history as outlined in **Table 1**. Although it does not specifically address the need to ask the patient about suicidal ideation, the Patient Health Questionnaire-9 (PHQ-2) is an ultrashort screener that can facilitate a conversation with the patient who may be at-risk for comorbid affective disorder.

### Posttraumatic Stress Disorder and Trauma

The essential features of PTSD follow direct experience of, or exposure to, one or several life-threatening events. Avoidant fear-based behaviors, depressed mood states, intrusive thoughts, heightened arousal, and panic encompass the core criteria. PTSD-related dissociative symptoms can be precipitated in a dental visit and are characterized by disrupted memory, a sense of being detached, and a distorted perception of the environment. Some patients commonly experience flashbacks and severe fear and avoidance associated with trigging events. About 3.6% of US adults experience a 12-month course of PTSD with 6.8% lifetime prevalence.[8] Women are twice as likely to experience PTSD as men.[14,21–24] Historically, the exposure to violence correlates with greater drug abuse severity independent of other psychiatric disorders.[14,20–24] Within the PTSD population, there is a likelihood of a 25% to 50% cooccurrence with SUD.[24] Those with PTSD exhibit a 2- to 4-fold incidence of SUD when compared with the general population.[25] Similarly, patients diagnosed as having an opioid use disorder have a 42% increased chance of having cooccurring PTSD.[26] Complicating the issue in dental practice, this comorbid relationship is particularly strong in patients who present with chronic facial pain conditions.[27]

### Bipolar Disorders

Bipolar disorders are now considered a distinct psychiatric category from Mood Disorders, and they are referenced as frequency, severity, and duration of the patient's manic, hypomanic, and depressive episodes.[8] This disorder is relevant for discussion in the context of dental practice, because 92% of people diagnosed with bipolar disorder have another comorbid psychiatric condition, most likely an SUD; this places bipolar disorders and SUDs among the highest of concomitant psychiatric disorder presentations.[28,29] Comorbid anxiety is also present in three-fourths of all cases. Although bipolar disorder impacts only 3% of the population, individuals with bipolar disorder carried out 25% of all completed suicides.[8,27] Alcohol and controlled substances are often involved during these suicide attempts. Given the above risk factors, the dentist is advised to better recognize this comorbid diagnosis because appropriate referral may have a great impact on the patient's well-being.

### Sleep Disorders

It is estimated that about 50 to 70 million Americans experience a sleep disorder.[30] As many as one-third of adults experience disruptive sleep symptoms and report insomnia, although only 6% to 10% of that population meets criteria for insomnia disorder.[8] Of those who experience clinical insomnia, 40% to 50% will experience another comorbid mental disorder. Depression, bipolar, and anxiety disorders are common comorbid conditions encountered for those with insomnia, and persistent insomnia elevates risk for developing an SUD. The presence of sleep disorders in children also may predict to later SUD risk.[31] With respect to comorbid SUD, parasomnias are of particular importance. These disorders are classified by disruptive motor behavior, nightmares, and disturbances in sleep and can be due to substance use and withdrawal. With the advent of dentistry now addressing obstructive sleep apnea, the widened scope of practice provides the field with an improved opportunity to recognize other common mental health comorbidities associated with sleep disorder, including comorbid SUD.

### Eating Disorders

Eating disorder mortalities are nearly twice as high compared with the general population and 6 times as high for those with anorexia nervosa.[32] Moreover, suicide rates in patients with eating disorders are 50 times higher compared with the general population. Those with a history of eating disorder are 2 to 4 times more likely to have an SUD when compared with the general population.[33] Given dentists' and dental hygienists' clinical skill in identifying eating disorders in general dental practice,[34] these clinicians may be in a unique position to identify and refer for management of comorbid SUDs.

## SOCIOECONOMIC, PSYCHOSOCIAL, AND RELATED DEMOGRAPHIC VARIABLES

There are several factors that can predict SUD, independent of psychiatric and medical risk indicators. For example, family history of substance abuse is a predictor of risk, as are financial hardship and unemployment. Interpersonal relationship factors can play a role, such a divorce or other unexpected changes in one's social supports. Chronic medical conditions can lead to loss of work, family, and social disruption, and loss of income, further increasing the risk for developing an SUD or relapse.[35]

Criminal behavior, such as diversion, doctor shopping to acquire multiple controlled substances, or forging prescriptions, is a difficult behavior to encounter for any dentist, and the presence of these issues might suggest active substance abuse by the offending patient. Fortunately, in cases where crimes have been alleged, involvement in the court system does not necessarily predict poor outcome with respect to the effectiveness of SUD treatment. The term "therapeutic jurisprudence" is used whereby SUD treatment may be mandated by the court. There are cases whereby mandated care results in longer treatment stays and better patient outcomes. Keith and colleagues[36] recently discussed these issues in a paper coauthored by a law-enforcement expert, suggesting that there may be a role for better collaboration where criminal behavior is discovered.

### Mental Status and Substance Abuse

Although details on mental status examination are beyond the scope of this article, a patient's inability to pay attention, understand dental care instructions, or recall recent and past events can be an immediate indicator of substance misuse or abuse. Cognitive impairments are also not exclusive to acute symptoms of alcohol abuse or withdrawal, and mental status changes should always be considered an indicator of substance abuse or misuse with other comorbid acute medical disorders. The use of brief mental status screeners has been addressed in the dental education literature, although training in this area remains lacking.[13,37]

## COMORBID MEDICAL CONDITIONS WITH SUBSTANCE ABUSE

Conducting a thorough patient history, physical examination, review of records, and conversation with cotreating medical providers offers the best step toward identifying medical comorbidities that may suggest the presence of an SUD. **Box 2** outlines the more common diseases and conditions associated with an increased substance abuse risk.[37]

While no single medical or psychiatric condition exclusively predicts a current substance use problem or risk of developing an SUD, the presence of specific medical conditions should alert the dentist to conduct a more thorough SUD risk assessment.

---

**Box 2**
**Common comorbid medical risk factors associated with substance abuse**

- Cerebrovascular disease
- Chronic renal and pulmonary disease
- Heart failure
- Nonmalignant pancreatic disease
- Obstructive sleep apnea
- Recurrent or chronic headache

---

For example, alcohol use disorder is associated with an increased risk in cerebral hemorrhages, dilated cardiomyopathy, hypertension, arrhythmias, peripheral artery disease, and death-associated acute cardiovascular (CV) events. Among a sample of 73 patients with heart failure, Tully and associates[38] found that 17.8% had a history of alcohol abuse or substance abuse.

Habitual smoking is also regarded as a risk factor for peripheral artery disease.[34] Smoking has also been associated with a higher risk of ischemia and cerebral hemorrhages.[39] Although the presence of pulmonary disease in a patient does not guarantee that they have a history as a tobacco smoker, there is a case to be made that those with pulmonary disease are more likely than not to have smoked or currently abuse tobacco. Tobacco use is causally linked with 80% to 90% of lung cancer deaths in the United States, with tobacco smoking accounting for 8 of 10 congestive obstructive pulmonary disease (COPD) deaths. Nearly 75% of Americans with COPD have a history of tobacco smoking.[40] A dental clinician who encounters a patient with pulmonary disease can establish a more accurate substance use history if they investigate specific tobacco use patterns among these patients.

Some CV disorders may also be associated with SUD, and one of the most common causes of dilated cardiomyopathy is alcohol use disorder. Stimulant and opioid use also may be associated with an increase in CV disease. In a study of 4800 active drug users, 223 were hospitalized because of CV disease. 1 in 5 adults aged 18 to 44 who experienced stroke had abused substances, and the drugs that have been most strongly associated with CV disease are stimulants and opioids.[41] Rios La Rosa and associates[42] conclude that adults under the age of 55 who have suffered a stroke should be routinely screened for SUD, another opportunity for providing improved assessment for geriatric dental patients.

With the rise of the opioid epidemic, there has also been an increase in the amount of infectious disease cases, in part because of intravenous (IV) drug use.[42] Using IV as the route of administration can directly affect the heart by causing infective endocarditis, which if not treated, can lead to stroke and heart attack. This risk is elevated if the patient has longstanding opioid use. Hepatitis C, a viral infection commonly found in IV drug users, may also have some association with some types of cardiomyopathy.[43]

The presence of liver function abnormalities in substance abusers should not be an overlooked risk factor. Steatohepatitis, alcohol hepatitis, and a liver cirrhosis diagnosis in the patient's medical history remain indicators for the presence of SUD. The dentist may discover the presence of these medical comorbidities by patient self-report, or upon receiving laboratory results or prior medical records. Follow-up with more thorough assessment is warranted.

## History of External Injuries and Emergency Department Visits

Even frequent visits to emergency departments (ED) can be a predictor of substance abuse, with as many as half of emergency room visits related to diagnoses of SUD.[44] EDs often see patients with common comorbid medical issues, including pulmonary disease, CV disease, gastrointestinal disease, and chronic headache. When facial injuries and other acute trauma are present, screening for domestic violence should always be addressed first. However, further assessment for substance use risk likewise requires serious consideration. Although other confounding socioeconomic factors, such as job loss, may predict higher frequency of ED visits, it is well established that patients who have frequent ED visits for pain, headache, or psychiatric disorders may be at higher risk for SUD and require judicious screening.

## SUMMARY

Navigating how to best evaluate and manage patients with controlled substance comorbid risks remains a complicated task. In clinical practice, the odds of encountering a patient without risk factors remain high, and the dental practitioner is now being tasked with these new responsibilities. With cost-effective screening strategies outlined in this series, dentists are in a better position to assess the patient, collaborate with cotreating health care providers, and manage the patient with risk for an SUD.

## DISCLOSURE

The authors have received funding grants (STUDY00000083) from the RIZE foundation. Partial support was received for the preparation of this article through a grant from "The Coverys Community Healthcare Foundation".

## REFERENCES

1. Häggman-Henrikson B, Ekberg E, Ettlin DA, et al. Mind the gap: a systematic review of implementation of screening for psychological comorbidity. J Dent Hyg 2018;82:1065–76.
2. Huntley AL, Johnson R, Purdy S, et al. Measures of multimorbidity and morbidity burden for use in primary care and community settings: a systematic review and guide. Ann Fam Med 2012;10(2):134–41.
3. Valderas JM, Starfield B, Sibbald B, et al. Defining comorbidity: implications for understanding health and health services. Ann Fam Med 2009;7(4):357–63.
4. Marpaung C, Lobbezoo F, Maurits S. Temporomandibular disorders among Dutch adolescents: prevalence and biological, psychological, and social risk indicators. Pain Res Manage 2018;2018:5053709.
5. Bartley E, Schmidt J, Carlson C, et al. Psychosocial considerations in TMD. In Temporomandibular Disorders. Basal, Switzerland: Springer International Publishing; 2018. p. 193–217.
6. Kisely S, Baghaie H, Lalloo R, et al. A systematic review and meta-analysis of the association between poor oral health and severe mental illness. Psychosom Med 2015;77(1):83–92.
7. Cleveland MJ, Feinberg ME, Bontempo DE, et al. The role of risk and protective factors in substance use across adolescence. J Adolesc Health 2008;43(2):157–64.
8. American Psychiatric Association. Diagnostic and statistical manual of mental disorders, fifth edition. Arlington (VA): American Psychiatric Association; 2013.

9. Substance Abuse and Mental Health Services Administration. Key substance use and mental health indicators in the United States: results from the 2018 National Survey on Drug Use and Health (HHS publication No. PEP19-5068, NSDUH series H-54). Rockville (MD): Center for Behavioral Health Statistics and Quality, Substance Abuse and Mental Health Services Administration; 2019.

10. Hjorthøj C, Østergaard ML, Benros ME, et al. Association between alcohol and substance use disorders and all-cause and cause specific mortality in schizophrenia, bipolar disorder, and unipolar depression: a nationwide, prospective, register-based study. Lancet Psychiatry 2015;2(9):801–8.

11. Grant BF, Saha TD, Ruan WJ, et al. Epidemiology of DSM-5 drug use disorder: results from the National Epidemiologic Survey on alcohol and related conditions–III. JAMA Psychiatry 2016;73(1):39–47.

12. Stoychev KR. Neuroimaging studies in patients with mental disorder and co-occurring substance use disorder: summary of findings. Front Psychiatry 2019; 10:702.

13. Kulich R, Backstrom J, Brownstein J, et al. A model for opioid risk stratification: assessing the psychosocial components of orofacial pain. Oral Maxillofac Surg Clin North Am 2016;28(3):261–73.

14. Back SE, Waldrop AE, Brady KT. Treatment challenges associated with comorbid substance use and posttraumatic stress disorder: clinicians' perspectives. Am J Addict 2009;18:15–20.

15. Dowell D, Haegerich TM, Chou R. CDC guideline for prescribing opioids for chronic pain—United States, 2016. MMWR Recomm Rep 2016;65:1–49.

16. Bandelow B, Michaelis S. Epidemiology of anxiety disorders in the 21st century. Dialogues Clin Neurosci 2015;17(3):327–35.

17. National Institute of Mental Health. Available at: https://www.nimh.nih.gov/health/statistics/any-anxiety-disorder.shtml. Accessed December 15, 2019.

18. Brownell K, Gold M. Food and addiction. New York: Oxford University Press; 2012.

19. Moscati A, Flint J, Kendler KS. Classification of anxiety disorders comorbid with major depression: common or distinct influences on risk. Depress Anxiety 2016; 33(2):120–7.

20. DeVeaugh- Geiss AM, West SL, Miller WC, et al. The adverse effects of comorbid pain on depression outcomes in primary care patients: results from the ARTIST trial. Pain Med 2010;11:732–41.

21. Institute of Medicine. Treatment for posttraumatic stress disorder in military and veteran populations: final assessment. Washington, DC: National Academies Press (US); 2014.

22. Khoury L, Tang YL, Bradley B, et al. Substance use, childhood traumatic experience, and posttraumatic stress disorder in an urban civilian population. Depress Anxiety 2010;27(12):1077–86.

23. Olff M. Sex and Gender Differences in Post Traumatic Stress Disorder: An Update. Eur J of psychotraumatol. 2017;8.

24. Banerjee S, Spry C. Concurrent treatment for substance use disorder and trauma-related comorbidities: a review of clinical effectiveness and guidelines 2017. Available at: https://www.ncbi.nlm.nih.gov/books/NBK525683/. Accessed December 15, 2019.

25. Gradus JL. Prevalence and prognosis of stress disorders: a review of the epidemiologic literature. Clin Epidemiol 2017;9:251–60.

26. Bilevicius E, Sommer JL, Asmundson GJG, et al. Posttraumatic stress disorder and chronic pain are associated with opioid use disorder: results from a 2012–

2013 American nationally representative survey. Drug Alcohol Depend 2018;188: 119–25.

27. Saunders EC, McGovern MP, Lambert-Harris C, et al. The impact of addiction medications on treatment outcomes for persons with co-occurring PTSD and opioid use disorders. Am J Addict 2015;24(8):722–31.

28. Salloum IM, Brown ES. Management of comorbid bipolar disorder and substance use disorders. Am J Drug Alcohol Abuse 2017;43(4):366–76.

29. National Institute for Mental Health. Bipolar disorder. 2017. Available at: https:// www.nimh.nih.gov/health/statistics/bipolar-disorder.shtml. Accessed January 02, 2020.

30. Yong LC, Li J, Calvert GM. Sleep-related problems in the US working population: prevalence and association with shiftwork status. Occup Environ Med 2017;74: 93–104.

31. Fortuna LR, Cook B, Porche MV, et al. Sleep disturbance as a predictor of time to drug and alcohol use treatment in primary care. Sleep Med 2018;42:31–7.

32. Schmidt U, Adan R, Bohm I, et al. Eating disorders: the big issue. Lancet Psychiatry 2016;3:313–5.

33. Steinberg B. Medical and dental implications of eating disorders. J Dent Hyg 2014;88(3):156–9.

34. Frimenk K, Murdoch-Kinch C, Inglehart M. Educating dental students about eating disorders. Perceptions and practice of interprofessional care. J Dent Educ 2017;81:1327–37.

35. Webster L. Risk factors for opioid-use disorder and overdose. Anesth Analg 2017;125(5):2017.

36. Keith D, Shannon T, Kulich R. The prescription monitoring program data: what it can tell you. J Am Dent Assoc 2018;149(4):266–72.

37. Webster L. Risk factors for opioid use and overdose. Anesthesia and Analgesia 2017;125(5):1741–8.

38. Tully PJ, Wittert G, Selkow T, et al. The real world mental health needs of heart failure patients are not reflected by the depression randomized controlled trial evidence. PLoS One 2014;9(1):e85928.

39. Pineda JR, Kim ES, Osinbowale OO. Impact of pharmacologic interventions on peripheral artery disease. Prog Cardiovasc Dis 2015;57(5):510–20.

40. Kaplan E, Gottesman R, Llinas R, et al. The association between specific substances of abuse and subcortical intracerebral hemorrhage versus ischemic lacunar infarction. Front Neurol 2014;5:174.

41. Centers for Disease Control and Prevention. Smoking and COPD 2019. Available at: https://www.cdc.gov/tobacco/campaign/tips/diseases/copd.html. Accessed December 16, 2019.

42. De los Ríos F, Kleindorfer DO, Khoury J, et al. Trends in substance abuse preceding stroke among young adults: a population-based study. Stroke 2012;43: 3179–83.

43. Onyeka IN, Beynon CM, Uosukainen H, et al. Coexisting social conditions and health problems among clients seeking treatment for illicit drug use in Finland: the HUUTI study. BMC Public Health 2013;13:380.

44. Substance Abuse and Mental Health Services Administration, Center for Behavioral Health Statistics and Quality. The DAWN report: highlights of the 2010 Drug Abuse Warning Network (DAWN) findings on drug-related emergency department visits. Rockville (MD): Center for Behavioral Health Statistics and Quality; 2012.

45. National Institute on Drug Abuse. Resource guide: screening for drug use in general medical settings 2012. Available at: https://www.drugabuse.gov/publications/resource-guide-screening-drug-use-in-general-medical-settings. Accessed January 01, 2020.

46. Rutter LA, Brown TA. Psychometric properties of the Generalized Anxiety Disorder Scale (GAD-7) in outpatients with anxiety and mood disorders. J Psychopathol Behav Assess 2017;39:140–6.

47. Connor K, Davidson J. SPRINT: a brief global assessment of post-traumatic stress disorder. Int Clin Psychopharmacol 2001;16:279–84.

48. Manea L, Gilbody S, Hewitt C, et al. Identifying depression with the PHQ-2: a diagnostic meta-analysis. J Affect Disord 2016;203:382–95.

# Assessment and Management of the High-Risk Dental Patient with Active Substance Use Disorder

Archana Viswanath, BDS, MS[a,b], Antje M. Barreveld, MD[c,d],
Matthew Fortino, MA[e,f],*

## KEYWORDS

- Brief intervention • Naloxone • Overdose • Prescreen • Referral • SBIRT
- Screening • Substance use disorder

## KEY POINTS

- The dental provider plays a key role in the care of patients with substance use disorders, working in collaboration with other medical professionals to determine the appropriate level of care and necessary referrals to promote optimal access, support, and treatment.
- Screening, brief intervention, and referral to treatment (SBIRT) is an approach to delivering early intervention and treatment, providing a framework for dental providers to assess patients through the use of brief validated screening tools, communication to increase awareness and motivation toward change, and access to specialty care when appropriate.
- The frequency and severity of medical emergencies related to patients presenting with substance use disorder in dental settings can be mitigated through application of the SBIRT model.
- Nonjudgmental, destigmatized, and compassionate communication between patients and providers is necessary to establish a therapeutic alliance and effectively promote recovery and patient safety.

[a] Department of Oral and Maxillofacial Surgery, Tufts University School of Dental Medicine, 1 Kneeland Street, Boston, MA 02111, USA; [b] Department of Diagnostic Sciences, Tufts University School of Dental Medicine, 1 Kneeland Street, Boston, MA 02111, USA; [c] Department of Anesthesiology, Tufts University School of Medicine, 1 Kneeland Street, Boston, MA 02111, USA; [d] Pain Management Services, Substance Use Services, Newton-Wellesley Hospital, Newton, MA, USA; [e] Department of Diagnostic Sciences, Center for Pain Medicine, Tufts University School of Dental Medicine, 1 Kneeland Street, Boston, MA 02111, USA; [f] Department of Anesthesia, Critical Care and Pain Medicine, Harvard Medical School and Massachusetts General Hospital, Boston, MA, USA
* Corresponding author.
*E-mail address:* mfortino@mgh.harvard.edu

Dent Clin N Am 64 (2020) 547–558
https://doi.org/10.1016/j.cden.2020.02.004
0011-8532/20/© 2020 Elsevier Inc. All rights reserved.

## INTRODUCTION

Opioid prescribing by dental providers has decreased steadily since 2012, yet the shift in prescribing trends has fallen short of implementing a comprehensive screening and referral paradigm for patients at risk for misusing prescription or illicit opioids or patients with an active substance use disorder (SUD) or opioid use disorder (**Box 1**).[1–4] Furthermore, the integration of risk mitigation assessments and mental health referrals has not been widely implemented despite their utility in averting both high-risk prescribing and inadequate follow-up care. This situation exists in stark contrast to the resounding data that indicate the dental setting is an opportune platform to implement screens, deliver brief interventions, and provide appropriate referrals. Therefore, it is within the purview of dental practitioners not only to identify who is at risk of developing an SUD but also to treat and offer guidance to help patients navigate health care systems and effectively remove the barriers that interfere with their access to care.[5]

Dentists and dental hygienists play a critical role in the assessment and management of complex dental patients, and their role in opioid risk mitigation to date has been underemphasized.[6–8] Dental practitioners have enduring relationships with their patients and are in a strategic position to utilize brief standardized assessment approaches. For example, screening, brief intervention, and referral to treatment (SBIRT) is a comprehensive, integrated, public health approach to inform treatment planning by identifying patients at risk for SUD (or those engaging in risky alcohol and drug use). As reviewed in other articles in this issue, the National Institute on Drug Abuse Quick Screen and its integrated SBIRT assessment pathway advise dental practitioners to assist in screening, provide brief interventions (eg, 5–10 minutes), and refer to treatment.[9] Dentist practitioners already possess

---

**Box 1**
**American Dental Association, October 2005, "Statement on Provision of Dental Treatment for Patients with Substance Use Disorders"**

1. Dentists are urged to be aware of each patient's substance use history and to take this into consideration when planning treatment and prescribing medications.

2. Dentists are encouraged to be knowledgeable about SUDs—both active and in remission—in order to safely prescribe controlled substances and other medications to patients with these disorders.

3. Dentists should draw on their professional judgment in advising patients who are heavy drinkers to cut back and the users of illegal drugs to stop.

4. Dentists may want to be familiar with their community's treatment resources for patients with SUDs and be able to make referrals when indicated.

5. Dentists are encouraged to seek consultation with a patient's physician, when the patient has a history of alcoholism or other SUD.

6. Dentists are urged to be current in their knowledge of pharmacology, including content related to drugs of abuse; recognition of contraindications to the delivery of epinephrine-containing local anesthetics; safe prescribing practices for patients with SUDs—both active and in remission; and management of patient emergencies that may result from unforeseen drug interactions.

7. Dentists are obliged to protect patient confidentiality of substances abuse treatment information, in accordance with applicable state and federal law.

*From* American Dental Association. Statement on provision of dental treatment for patients with substance use disorders. Available at: https://www.ada.org/en/advocacy/current-policies/substance-use-disorders. Copyright © 2005 American Dental Association. All rights reserved. Reprinted with permission.

considerable knowledge of prescription opioids, because they provide treatment guided by established prescribing standards, which necessitate SUD risk assessment in managing acute pain. This article is designed to review the goals of assessment by defining the methodology relevant to the contributions of the entire dental team.

## IDENTIFYING SUBSTANCE USE DISORDER IN THE DENTAL PRACTICE

A detailed medical and psychosocial history is necessary to properly screen and identify a patient with a potential SUD. The medical history also must include a family history (including history of SUD) as well as current medications, smoking status (tobacco and cannabis), alcohol use, and illicit drug use, denoting both frequency and administration of the substance (vaped, injected, inhaled, and so forth). The type and method of administration of each substance may be important in identifying a patient's likelihood of contracting an infectious disease, risk of mental and physical health consequences, and adherence to treatment recommendations. Cicero and Ellis[10] observed how some, but not all, patients who orally administer opioids may move to other dosing routes like insufflation or intravenous injection, both delivery systems associated with increased exposure and vulnerability to infectious disease. In addition to infectious diseases, intravenous use is associated with a 100-times increased likelihood of developing deep vein thrombosis compared with the general population.[11]

The NM ASSIST (National Institute of Drug Abuse Modified Alcohol, Smoking, and Substance Involvement Screening Test) outline a more detailed investigation of drug use history if the results from the quick screen are positive; details on this screening approach are discussed in depth in other articles in this issue. Routine screening for alcohol use also should be performed using brief questionnaires, such as the AUDIT-C (Alcohol Use Disorder Identification Test for Consumption).[12] The CUDIT-R (Cannabis Use Disorder Identification Test-Revised) can query for problematic cannabis use, another area of increasing interest for clinicians concerned about oral health.[13,14]

Despite the availability of validated screening measures, stigmatizing factors related to substance use may have an impact on the accuracy of a patient's self-report. Social desirability bias, legal implications of admitting to illicit activities, and implicit cognitive process are factors that may cause a patient to deny or underreport use of a substance.[15,16] The risk of collecting unreliable self-report data belies the need for dentists to be aware of physical and oral manifestations of drug use.[6] There are several intraoral symptoms associated with substance use, such as rampant caries, poor oral hygiene, advanced periodontitis, xerostomia, a high percentage of missing teeth, traumatic lesions, and oral infection.[8,17–19] The opportunity for dentists to provide brief intervention and referral can arise from any dental encounter.[20] Common oral symptoms associated with substance use are listed in **Table 1**.

McNeely and associates[21] discuss various factors related to dentists recognizing an SUD. The implementation of screens and the referral to treatment services were limited, however, to alcohol and tobacco and not evenly distributed among dentists, depending on their geographic region. It was proposed that the disparity in perceived utility of screens and the scarce application of them lies not in dentist aptitude, but rather in the majority of training curriculums that fail to include clinical opportunities and practice-based systems focused on SUD that could facilitate patient-provider discussions, support, and access to treatment.

## BRIEF INTERVENTION AND BRIEF TREATMENT

The component of SBIRT that follows screening is brief intervention and/or brief treatment. This 20-fold process offers dental clinicians the opportunity to promote patients'

**Table 1**
**Intraoral findings commonly found in patients with commonly abused substances**

| Drug | Oral Manifestations |
|---|---|
| Alcohol | Oral mucosal discoloration<br>   Stomatitis: red atrophic oral mucosa; yellow-brown discoloration<br>   Glossodynia: atrophic red beefy tongue<br>Leukoplakia<br>Distinct halitosis (fruity acetone breadth)<br>Multiple caries and/or periodontal disease<br>Enlarged salivary glands (particularly parotid)<br>Xerostomia<br>Bruxism<br>Reduced tolerance to pain |
| Cannabis | Distinct greenish staining of tongue and oral cavity<br>Xerostomia<br>High risk for periodontal disease<br>   Gingival hyperplasia<br>   Alveolar bone loss<br>   Clinical periodontal attachment loss |
| Chronic opioid use | Clenching, bruxism<br>Xerostomia<br>Increased susceptibility to periodontitis and dental caries |
| Cocaine | Dyskinesia<br>Jerky movements of the face uncontrolled<br>Xerostomia<br>Gingival attachment loss (test for potency by rubbing on gingiva)<br>Bruxism |
| Heroin/fentanyl | Teeth erosion due to frequent vomiting? From withdrawal? |
| Methamphetamine | Extensive caries<br>Characteristic meth caries<br>Chelation reaction that cleaves enamel from dentin |

insight and awareness concerning their substance use in order to assist with behavioral change.[22,23] In this step, the goal for the dental practitioner is to educate patients and promote their motivation to reduce or stop the use of harmful substances. The dentist should ask for a patient's informal permission to receive feedback before advice is offered. Brief open-ended questions and motivational phrases may include, "Would you mind taking a few minutes to talk with me about your alcohol use?"; "Hello, I looked through your intake questionnaires. I'm worried about you. How are you doing?"; "I notice you have very advanced dental decay, which we may see with substance use. Could you talk with me about your health so that I can best support you?"; and "What connection do you see between your substance use and your dental findings?" To apply motivational interviewing principles, the dentist should try using language that acknowledges the autonomy of patients by emphasizing their personal choice. See **Box 2** for examples adapted from Miller and Rollnick.[24] The format provided allows dentists to offer several options for referrals or treatment recommendations, which can enhance a patient's experience of choice and collaboration. Good chairside manner and a compassionate team approach make dental procedures less harrowing for any patient.

Despite an empathic and therapeutic alliance, patients may disagree with their provider. Dentists should remain noncombative and validate patients' concerns before offering suggestions. **Table 2** provides the 7 Es, proposed by Becker and associates[25]

---

**Box 2**
**Autonomy supportive language prompts**

"In the end the decision is up to you, but I can describe some options if you'd like."

"You may or may not agree with this idea…"

"If you wish, you could try…"

"I can't tell you what to do, but I can tell you what's worked for other patients."

---

as a method of evoking awareness within a patient presenting with pain. It is up to dental professionals to decide how to connect the conversation style to their practice. The result may look something like this: "For some people, taking opioids daily can actually make pain worse. If it's all right with you, I can go over programs that have helped other patients manage their pain."

Advice is more likely to be acted on when there is a strong therapeutic alliance between provider and patient.[26] As the expert in the room, the dentist is in a position to share the reasons why and how a patient could change. How the dentist goes about this can facilitate the exchange of information. In practice, it is useful to have patients be their own expert and ask open-ended questions about what they know (substance in question) and what they would like to know. The dentist should consider what patients most wants or needs to know, and, after educating them, have them reiterate what has been advised in their own words. Through this collaborative process, the dental professional can provide patients with options and guide them to the next step in treatment.

## REFERRAL TO TREATMENT

Brief treatment is a more intensive procedure that typically is performed in an outpatient setting. Brief treatment morphs into the third SBIRT component, which is referral to an identified health professional or team to provide long-term, resource-intensive

---

**Table 2**
**Methods and demeanor to evoke awareness within the dental patient**

| 7 Es | Examples |
|---|---|
| 1. Express empathy | "I understand that you are in pain and that this is causing you significant anxiety and distress." |
| 2. Elicit functional goals | "What activities would you like to do that your pain is preventing you from doing?" |
| 3. Educate | "For some patients, continuous use of opioids can actually result in more pain by lowering the pain threshold." |
| 4. Endorse an alternative plan | "A lower dose of opioids may make you less sedated and allow you to improve your ability to do the activities you want to do." |
| 5. Enlist patient buy-in | "Would you be willing to try a lower dose of opioids or switch to a combination of nonopioid options? " |
| 6. Enact follow-up plan | "Would you be willing to meet every 2 weeks to discuss your progress?" |
| 7. Equanimity | Be calm, even-tempered, and nonjudgmental throughout the conversation |

treatment. Dental professionals are not expected to conduct these lengthy sessions themselves and are encouraged to coordinate care with SUD specialists and primary care. Although all patients can be referred for treatment, high-risk patients who test positive on the brief screens or meet criteria for an SUD always should be offered a referral. This process requires that the clinician coordinate care to bypass factors that may impede a patient's ability to access and engage treatment. This process may entail prescribing transportation services, following-up with a referral provider post–patient intake, and continuing communication with the treating provider.[27]

Gauging a patient's readiness for change and barriers for accessing treatment may help assist a team in following-up with a patient after a clinical encounter and help support the patient's next steps. Dentists have an ethical obligation to discuss concerns about substance use with their patients and direct them to an appropriate level of care. The American Dental Association (ADA) "Principles of Ethics and Code of Professional Conduct" declares, "dentists shall be obliged to seek consultation, if possible, whenever the welfare of patients will be safeguarded or advanced by using those who have special skills, knowledge, and experience.[23]

The referral process should be accessible to patients, and the dental office should have an established referral protocol in place. The referral base in the dental office should include, among others, pain management specialists, addiction specialists, psychiatrists, counseling services, and peer and family support resources. Resources for addiction services also should include state dental societies, local hospitals, and state governments. Electronic prescription drug monitoring programs also may provide a resource list of suitable providers that can be accessed directly from a patient's electronic data sheet. The Substance Abuse and Mental Health Services Administration (SAMHSA) may be consulted, for treatment and referral recommendations, as can the SAMHSA substance abuse treatment facility locator, which lists local community treatment centers and resources.[28]

When communicating with patients about a referral to a treatment program or substance use specialist, the practitioner should use the same manner and wording used to refer them to any other type of specialist:

1. Express and explain concerns to the patient.
2. Obtain patient consent to communicate with the referral provider.
3. Provide the patient with name of the referral and expertise, geographic location, and any possible charges associated with service.
4. Follow-up with the referring provider or patient to ensure care has been accessed.

## DENTAL MANAGEMENT OF PATIENTS WITH SUBSTANCE USE DISORDER

There are several challenges a dental professional may face when treating patients with an active SUD. A patient might experience comorbid anxiety or other mental illnesses contributing to varying cognitions like fear of pain alongside perceptions of loss of control. Additionally, a patient's pain tolerance may waver, further agitated by the anxiety of initiating or tapering from a longstanding medication regimen.[29] Patients with an SUD may be using multiple substances and are at a greater risk of suffering from comorbid psychiatric conditions.[30] Patients who meet criteria for SUD also may suffer from persistent problems of oral hygiene in addition to the effects of drugs on the oral cavity, as listed in **Table 1**.

It is important to account for active SUD when administering local anesthesia because every organ system is affected by the introduction of psychotropic drugs, and the impact of such chemicals can influence treatment in unpredictable ways.[31] Polysubstance use can lead to unexpected drug-drug interactions that may impart an additive, synergistic, or antagonistic effect to the medication efficacy.[32] Certain combinations can trigger adverse drug-induced events, which account for approximately one-third of all hospital adverse events in the United States.[33] To avoid such occurrences, note the frequently abused substances, discussed later, and their implications on anesthesia and other dental care.

## DRUGS OF MISUSE

With the legal status of cannabis under reconsideration in a growing number of US states, dentists can expect to encounter patients more frequently who use cannabis and its psychoactive derivatives. Data indicate that the cultural shift has led to increases in use among the general population as well as youth for both medical and recreational purposes.[34]

Chronic cannabis use may produce a prolonged decrease in heart rate and blood pressure. Patients who smoke cannabis may experience a sudden increase in sympathetic activity with reduction of parasympathetic activity, followed by reflex tachycardia.[35] As a result, heart rate increases to account for the ensuing drop in blood pressure.[36] Evidence suggests that there is risk for increased susceptibility to cardiac ischemia or angina due to the association of elevated cardiac activity and subsequent oxygen deficiency in the blood, which occurs on use of cannabinoids. Those with cardiovascular disease may be particularly vulnerable to health risks given associations of atrial fibrillation, consequent of increased cardiac output.[37,38] Disseminating this information can safeguard patients from sustaining unexpected injuries consequent of postural hypotension, dizziness, and syncope.[37]

Adverse events caused by cannabis increasingly are recognized as are drug interactions.[37] Absolute contraindications to cannabis use include acute psychosis, and relative contraindications include severe cardiovascular, immunologic, liver, and kidney disease.[39] The authors also advise that local anesthetics should be administered without epinephrine for patients with recent cannabis use, because there is a potential to induce persistent tachycardia with epinephrine. Concerning variations among users, some patients who use cannabis, in particular naïve users, may respond less favorably than others and require further monitoring. Route of administration also can attenuate risk, for example, vaping or smoking may demonstrate greater risk than some means of use.

Cocaine use is a serious concern in dentistry because chronic cocaine use leads to elevated health risks and higher rates of bleeding and hemorrhage after routine dental extractions. In chronic use, perforations of the nasal septum and palate are common.[40,41] Administration of local anesthetic is contraindicated in patients actively using cocaine because it increases the risk of convulsions.[42] Epinephrine also is contraindicated because it puts patients at risk for an acute rise in blood pressure, which potentially could lead to cardiac arrest.[41] General anesthesia, however, does not increase mortality risk for cocaine users provided they have normal cardiovascular function at the time of procedure.[43] If multiple dental procedures are needed for someone who chronically uses cocaine, general anesthesia is the safer alternative.[43] Cocaine use within 24 hours before dental treatment can increase the risk of cardiovascular complications, especially if local anesthesia is used. Dental procedures should be postponed if a patient presents with signs of cocaine use.

Opioids also are a concern and are discussed at length in other articles in this issue. Chronic fentanyl use is a rising health concern with respect to overdose risk, although heroin remains a problem, with approximately 500,000 individuals misusing this drug in the United States[44] and an estimated 2.1 million with opioid use disorder overall.[45]

Heroin and fentanyl, like other opioids, have the potential for dangerous interaction with many drugs used in dentistry. The most severe medical complication associated with opioid misuse is the risk of respiratory depression. Patients who misuse opioids experience euphoria, drowsiness, and respiratory depression and are more prone to syncope.[46]

Managing acute dental or postoperative pain in patients with opioid use disorder can be challenging for dentists, and nonopioid management should be maximized. In addition to immediate intoxication, opioid-induced hyperalgesia can occur in those who are exposed to long-term opioid use and is characterized by sensitization to pain caused by exposure to opioids.[3,4] This phenomenon is not limited to those with opioid use disorder and can occur in any individual prescribed long-term opioids for chronic cancer and noncancer pain.

Individuals using methamphetamine generally delay seeking dental treatment until the pain becomes critical, often receiving dental care in emergency settings. One study demonstrated that individuals using methamphetamine waited an average of 17 months to seek care despite the presence of bleeding gums and temporomandibular joint pain.[47] If methamphetamine use is suspected, extreme care is required in choice and administration of local anesthesia. Methamphetamine increases a patient's risk for irregular heartbeat, heart attacks, and stroke. Local anesthetics with vasoconstrictors may be ineffective in relieving a patient's pain and are contraindicated due to the potential cardiovascular risks. If local anesthetic is used, it is critical that the patient avoid using methamphetamines within the previous 24 hours. If deep sedation is required, methamphetamine use must be discontinued for several days prior to the appointment.[48,49] On the day of the appointment, the dental team should observe the patient's behavior for possible symptoms of methamphetamine use or use reliable screening techniques to avoid the possibility of adverse drug interactions.[50]

## HOW TO PREPARE DENTAL PRACTICE FOR A SUBSTANCE USE EMERGENCY

The ADA Council on Dental Practice, with support from the ADA Health Policy Institute, conducted the "Survey on Preparedness for Medical Emergencies in the Dental Practice" in 2018.[51] The purpose of the survey was to assess preparedness for medical emergencies that could occur in the dental practice. The top 3 medical emergencies occurring in dental practices during the 12 months prior to the survey were syncope (39.77%), epinephrine reaction (37.43%), and postural hypotension (33.92%). Approximately 97% of all dental practices reported having a plan for responding to medical emergencies.

Given widespread controlled substance use and abuse, it is prudent for dentists to review training procedures and update their emergency kits to respond appropriately in the setting of a patient opioid overdose. The Centers for Disease Control and Prevention recommend that all health care providers are prepared to administer naloxone (the life-saving opioid reversal medication) to patients who are at risk for overdose,[43] and there are specific controlled substance risk/naloxone administration training programs reviewed elsewhere in this issue. Furthermore, most states have laws designed to protect health care professionals from civil and criminal liabilities to prescribe, dispense, and administer naloxone during an opioid overdose emergency.[52,53]

Naloxone is a fast-acting drug that can be administered, via an intramuscular injection or intranasal spray, to temporarily reverse the effects of an opioid overdose. Because the effects last only between 20 minutes and 90 minutes, an overdose may recur. When an opioid overdose is suspected, 911 always should be contacted to activate emergency medical services at the time of the overdose. It is recommended that dentists obtain naloxone for emergency use and receive appropriate training, and some states have mandated coprescribing naloxone if a dentist prescribes an opioid, 50 morphine milligram equivalents or greater, or concurrently prescribed high-risk substances, such as benzodiazepines.[54] Proper training includes education related to recognizing opioid overdose, administering naloxone, and remaining current with training for basic life support and cardiopulmonary resuscitation.

In summary, the dental provider should play a key role in the care of patients with SUDs, working in collaboration with other medical professionals to determine the appropriate level of care and necessary referrals to promote optimal access, support, and treatment. SBIRT is an effective approach to delivering early intervention and treatment, providing a framework for dental providers to assess patients through the use of brief validated screening tools, communication to increase awareness and motivation toward change, and access to specialty care when appropriate. The frequency and severity of SUD-related medical emergencies in dental settings can be mitigated through SBIRT. Finally, because dentists encounter these patients a regular basis, nonjudgmental, destigmatized, and compassionate communication between patients and providers is necessary to establish a therapeutic alliance and effectively promote recovery and patient safety.

## DISCLOSURE

The authors received funding grant (STUDY00000083) from the RIZE foundation. Partial support was received for the preparation of this article through a grant from "The Coverys Community Healthcare Foundation".

## REFERENCES

1. Tran BX, Moir M, Latkin CA, et al. Global research mapping of substance use disorder and treatment 1971–2017: implications for priority setting. Subst Abuse Treat Prev Policy 2019;14:21.
2. US Opioid Prescribing Rate Maps. Available at: https://www.cdc.gov/drugoverdose/maps/rxrate-maps.html. Accessed January 1, 2020.
3. Berna C, Kulich RJ, Rathmell JP. Tapering long-term opioid therapy in chronic noncancer pain: evidence and recommendations for everyday practice. Mayo Clin Proc 2015;90:828–84.
4. Kulich RJ, Backstrom J, Brownstein J, et al. A model for opioid risk stratification. Oral Maxillofac Surg Clin North Am 2016;28(3):261–73.
5. Atchison K, Weintraub J, Rozier R. Bridging the dental medical divide. J Am Dent Assoc 2018;149:850–8.
6. Centore L, Reisner L, Pettengill CA. Better understanding your patient from a psychological perspective: early identification of problem behaviors affecting the dental office. J Am Dent Assoc 2002;30:512–9.
7. Wentworth RB. What should I do when I suspect a patient may be abusing prescription drugs? J Am Dent Assoc 2008;139:623–4.
8. Newman CC, Bolton LW. Substance abuse and the dental patient. What's the connection? Dent Assist 2003;72:14–9.
9. Pervanas HC, Landry E, Southard DR, et al. Assessment of Screening, Brief Intervention, and Referral to Treatment Training to Interprofessional Health-Care Students. SAGE Open Nursing 2019;5:1–7.

10. Cicero T, Ellis M. Oral and non-oral routes of administration among prescription opioid users: Pathways, decision-making and directionality. Addict Behav 2018; 86:11–6.
11. Rauck RL. Mitigation of IV abuse through the use of abuse-deterrent opioid formulations: an overview of current technologies. Pain Pract 2019;19(4):443–54.
12. Khadjesari Z, White IR, McCambridge J, et al. Validation of the AUDIT-C in adults seeking help with their drinking online. Addict Sci Clin Pract 2017;12:2.
13. Annaheim B, Legleve S. Chapter 17 - Short instruments to screen for "problematic" cannabis use in general population surveys. In: Preedy VR, editor. Handbook of cannabis and related pathologies. Biology, pharmacology, diagnosis and treatment. London: Academic Press; 2017. p. 168–84.
14. Yudko E, Lozhkina O, Fouts A. A comprehensive review of the psychometric properties of the drug abuse screening test. J Subst Abuse Treat 2007;32(2): 189–98.
15. Clark CB, Zyambo CM, Li Y, et al. The impact of non-concordant self-report of substance use in clinical trials research. Addict Behav 2016;58:74–9.
16. Parish CL, Pereyra MR, Pollack HA, et al. Screening for substance misuse in the dental care setting: findings from a nationally representative survey of dentists. Addiction 2015;110(9):1516–23.
17. Da Fonseca MA. Substance use disorder in adolescence: a review for the pediatric dentist. J Dent Child 2009;76:209–16.
18. Shetty V, Mooney LJ, Zigler CM, et al. The relationship between methamphetamine use and increased dental disease. J Am Dent Assoc 2010;141:307–18.
19. Fung EY, Giannini PJ. Implications of drug dependence on dental patient management. Gen Dent 2010;58:236–41.
20. Solaiman T. RM matters: drug seekers—protect yourself from patients who abuse pain medications. Northwest Dent 2010;89:55–6.
21. McNeely J, Wright S, Matthews AG, et al. Substance-use screening and interventions in dental practices: Survey of practice-based research network dentists regarding current practices, policies and barriers. JAMA 2013;144:627–38.
22. McCance-Katz EF, Satterfield J. SBIRT: a key to integrate prevention and treatment of substance abuse in primary care. Am J Addict 2012;21(2):176–7.
23. American Dental Association. Principles of ethics and code of professional conduct. Available at: https://www.ada.org/~/media/ADA/Member%20Center/Ethics/Code_Of_Ethics_Book_With_Advisory_Opinions_Revised_to_November_2018.pdf?la=en. Accessed December 1, 2019.
24. Miller W, Rollnick S. Motivational interviewing. 3rd edition. New York: Guilford Press; 2013.
25. Becker WC, Merlin JS, Manhapra A, et al. Management of patients with issues related to opioid safety and/or misuse: a case series from an integrated, interdisciplinary clinic. Addict Sci Clin Pract 2016;11(1):3.
26. Lebow L. Couple and family therapy: an integrative map of the territory. Washington, DC: APA; 2014.
27. Substance Abuse and Mental Health Services Administration. Systems-level implementation of screening, brief intervention, and referral to treatment. Rockville (MD): Substance Abuse and Mental Health Services Administration; 2013. Technical Assistance Publication (TAP) Series 33. HHS Publication No. (SMA) 13-4741.
28. SAMHSA. Behavioral Health Treatment Services Locator2019. Available at: https://findtreatment.samhsa.gov/. Accessed December 1, 2019.
29. Freeman RE. Dental anxiety: a multifactorial aetiology. Br Dent J 1985;159:406–8.

30. Stoychev KR. Neuroimaging studies in patients with mental disorder and co-occurring substance use disorder: summary of findings. Front Psychiatry 2019; 10:702.

31. Hernandez M, Birnbach DJ, Zundert AAV. Anesthetic management of the illicit-substance-using patient. Curr Opin Anaesthesiol 2005;18:315–24.

32. Alsherbiny MA, Li CG. Medicinal cannabis-potential drug interactions. Medicines (Basel) 2018;6(1):3.

33. Office of Disease and Health Promotion. Adverse drug events. Available at: https://health.gov/hcq/ade.asp. Accessed December 1, 2019.

34. DiBenedetto DJ, Weed VF, Wawrzyniak KM, et al. The association between cannabis use and aberrant behaviors during chronic opioid therapy for chronic pain. Pain Med 2018;19(10):1997–2008.

35. Patel R, Manocha P, Patel J, et al. Cannabis use is an independent predictor for acute myocardial infarction related hospitalization in younger population. J Adolesc Health 2020;66:79–85.

36. Goyal H, Awad HH, Ghali JK. Role of cannabis in cardiovascular disorders. J Thorac Dis 2017;9(7):2079–92.

37. Korantzopoulos P, Liu T, Papaioannides D, et al. Atrial fibrillation and marijuana smoking. Int J Clin Pract 2008;62(2):308–31.

38. Russo E, MacCallum C. Practical considerations in medical cannabis administration and dosing. Eur J Intern Med 2018;49:12–9.

39. Government of District of Columbia Department of Health. Medical cannabis adverse effects and drug interactions. Available at: https://doh.dc.gov/sites/default/files/dc/sites/doh/publication/attachments/Medical%20Cannabis%20Adverse%20Effects%20and%20Drug%20Interactions_0.pdf. Accessed January 1, 2020.

40. Quart AM, Small CB, Klein RS. The cocaine connection. Users imperil their gingiva. JAMA 1991;122:85–7.

41. Lange RA, Hillis LD. Cardiovascular complications of cocaine use. N Engl J Med 2001;345(5):351.

42. Yagiela JA. Adverse drug interactions in dental practice: interactions associated with vasoconstrictors. Part V of a series. JAMA 1999;130:701–9.

43. Hill GE, Ogunnaike BO. Johnson ER general anaesthesia for the cocaine abusing patient. Is it safe? Br J Anaesth 2006;97(5):654–7.

44. Dowell D, Haegerich TM, Chou R. CDC guideline for prescribing opioids for chronic pain - United States, 2016. MMWR Recomm Rep 2016;65(1):1–49. Available at: https://www.cdc.gov/drugoverdose/prescribing/guideline.html.

45. Abraham A, Andrews C, Harris S, et al. Availability of medications for the treatment of alcohol and opioid use disorder in the USA. Neurotherpaeutics 2020; 17(1):55–69.

46. Cook H, Peoples J, Paden M. Management of the oral surgery patient addicted to heroin. J Oral Maxillofac 1989;47:281–5.

47. National Institute on Drug Abuse. Research Report Series: methamphetamine Abuse and Addiction. The relationship between methamphetamine use and increased dental disease. Bethesda (MD): National Institutes of Health; 2002. NIH Publication No. 02-4210.

48. McGee SM, McGee DN, McGee MB. Spontaneous intracerebral hemorrhage related to methamphetamine abuse: autopsy findings and clinical correlation. Am J Forensic Med Pathol 2004;25:334–7.

49. Howe AM. Methamphetamine and childhood and adolescent caries. Aust Dent J 1995;40(5):340.

50. Goodchild JH, Donaldson M. Methamphetamine abuse and dentistry: a review of the literature and presentation of a clinical case. Quintessence Int 2007;38: 583–90.
51. ADA survey on preparedness for medical emergencies in the dental practice. 2018. Available a: https://success.ada.org/en/practice-management/patients/2018-survey-on-preparedness-for-medical-emergencies. Accessed December 3, 2019.
52. Prescription drug abuse policy system, naloxone overdose prevention laws, 2017. Available at: www.pdaps.org. Accessed December 3, 2019.
53. National Association of State Alcohol and Drug Abuse Directors. Single State Agency for substance abuse: Resource to check third party prescription laws and Good Samaritan laws. Available at: http://nasadad.org/ssa-web-sites/. Accessed December 3, 2019.
54. Jones CM, Compton W, Vythilingam M, et al. Naloxone co-prescribing to patients receiving prescription opioids in the medicare part D program, United States, 2016-2017. JAMA 2019;322(5):462–4.

# Brief Motivational Interventions
## Strategies for Successful Management of Complex, Nonadherent Dental Patients

Michael E. Schatman, PhD[a,b,*], Hannah Shapiro[c],
María F. Hernández-Nuño de la Rosa, DDS, MS[d],
Vanak Huot, RDH, MPH[e]

KEYWORDS

• Motivational interviewing • dental settings • substance abuse

KEY POINTS

• Motivational interviewing (MI) is an evidence-based approach to resolving patient ambivalence to change.
• MI techniques can be effectively used by dentists in assessing and managing substance use risk and may add minimal time to the patient interview.
• Although MI's greatest utility has been in the area of improving general oral hygiene in order to reduce caries and other preventable conditions, its use in addressing controlled substance risk is well established in other health care disciplines.
• These techniques do not require special training in mental health assessment and can be effectively used by dentists and dental hygienists.

## INTRODUCTION

Motivational interviewing (MI) has been used in various forms in dental medicine for more than 20 years, with a review of the literature indicating that its applications have focused to a greater extent on general dental health than on substance misuse and abuse issues. This focus on the use of MI primarily for issues of general oral health is not surprising, because much of oral health (eg, prevention of pediatric cares) is

[a] Department of Diagnostic Sciences, Tufts University School of Dental Medicine, 1 Kneeland Street, Boston, MA 02111, USA; [b] Department of Public Health & Community Medicine, Tufts University School of Medicine, Boston, MA, USA; [c] Department of Biopsychology, Tufts University, Robinson Hall, 200 College Avenue, Medford, MA 02155, USA; [d] Department of Diagnostic Sciences, Craniofacial Pain and Sleep Center, Tufts University School of Dental Medicine, 1 Kneeland Street, Boston, MA 02111, USA; [e] Department of Clinical Affairs, Tufts University School of Dental Medicine, 1 Kneeland Street, Boston, MA 02111, USA
* Corresponding author. Department of Diagnostic Sciences, Tufts University School of Dental Medicine, Boston, MA.
*E-mail address:* michael.schatman@tufts.edu

Dent Clin N Am 64 (2020) 559–569
https://doi.org/10.1016/j.cden.2020.02.005
0011-8532/20/© 2020 Elsevier Inc. All rights reserved.

contingent on self-management,[1] with a 2016 systematic review[2] concluding that oral health education for patients is provided most effectively within the context of an MI approach. Several studies and reviews have concluded that MI training in general dentistry results in improved oral health and oral health knowledge,[3,4] and recent research indicates that MI training is progressively being successfully integrated into undergraduate and postgraduate dental and dental hygiene training.[5–7] The ultimate goal is to provide dentists and dental hygienists with the professional communication and listening skills required to achieve trusting relationships with patients before the completion of their training. This goal will allow them to enhance history taking as well as treatment planning and thus to provide the appropriate dental health care in a setting of a nationwide substance use crisis.

## ALCOHOL ABUSE

Given that MI has its roots in addiction treatment, some of the earlier clinical applications and empirical investigations of the efficacy of MI in dentistry pertained to reducing the use of potentially dangerous substances. An early review by Smith and colleagues[8] addressed the benefits of an MI approach to patients with maxillofacial pain who were traumatically injured while intoxicated by alcohol. The investigators noted that many of these patients were binge drinkers and were not particularly amenable to more direct behavioral change approaches. They noted that those with facial injuries were often overwhelmed by feelings of vulnerability, so clinic visits presented an opportune setting and time for brief MI interventions, because the patients' vulnerability enhanced readiness to change. Smith and colleagues[8] were not grandiose in their experiences and expectations, suggesting that such an approach would require only a brief amount of time to implement, and that perhaps 10% of such patients would alter their self-destructive drinking behavior consequently. A more recent study of MI for dental patients with alcohol-related facial trauma[9] in which behavioral intervention was provided by nurses yielded encouraging results. At 12 months post-intervention, those patients who received brief MI had reduced their alcohol consumption significantly more than the control group, which received educational pamphlets on alcohol misuse. In addition, a 2017 narrative review[10] determined that an abridged form of MI that the investigators called a brief alcohol intervention is effective in reducing reinjury occurrence and modifying alcohol intake, and recommended that patients with alcohol-related facial injury presenting to emergency departments should be treated with such interventions.

In addition to studies of the efficacy of MI for prevention of alcohol-related facial injuries, there exists a robust body of empirical literature supporting MI for alcohol abuse generally. Further, there is literature emphasizing the need for dentists to screen for alcohol abuse for purposes of oral cancer prevention. A 2006 study[11] found that more than 75% of dental patients approved of dentists screening and counseling regarding inappropriate consumption of alcohol. However, irrespective of the formidable body of literature in medicine and psychology supporting MI for the treatment of hazardous drinking more generally,[12–16] studies have not addressed this treatment approach in the dental literature. This omission may be caused by dentists' senses of embarrassment and perceived incompetence in addressing problematic alcohol use, despite their beliefs that doing so is beneficial to their patients.[17] Neff and colleagues[18] performed a comprehensive review of all articles published in the *Journal of the American Dental Association*, *Journal of Dental Education*, and the *Journal of Public Health Dentistry* between 1980 and 2010, finding that a total of only 2 articles addressing alcohol cessation counseling (both in the *Journal of the American Dental Association*) were published during this 30-year period. Neither of these articles[19,20] makes any mention of MI. However, since 2011, an empirical investigation of MI in dental settings for reducing alcohol consumption has appeared. Neff and colleagues[21] developed and applied a screening and brief intervention protocol (a principal component of which was MI) in a cluster-randomized trial to successfully reduce consumption quantity and frequency of alcohol use. Dental providers should be comfortable screening patients for potential alcohol use disorder and be prepared to recognize the most common general warning signs associated with alcohol abuse, such as irritability and/or extreme mood changes, isolation from friends and family members, or drinking alcohol to deal with stress, as well as the usual oral red flags such as poor oral hygiene and high prevalence of caries and periodontal disease. If these signs are present, the dentist or dental hygienist should take action accordingly and refer the patient to a local substance use specialist immediately. Appropriate motivational interview strategies facilitate a fluid communication based in mutual respect and appreciation between the dental provider and the patient, which helps more effectively address any potential substance use issues that might exist.

## TOBACCO USE

Numerous studies of MI in dentistry relating to smoking cessation appear in the literature. An early study was published by Koerber and colleagues,[22] in which the investigators found that dental student training in brief MI resulted in students using more brief MI techniques in their counseling of patients regarding smoking cessation. A more recent article[23] on integrating smoking cessation advice and support into daily dental practice highlighted the need for training dentists in MI. When combined with brief advice, MI in the dental setting has been shown to promote smoking cessation.[24] Although the randomized controlled trial did not address smoking, per se, Severson and colleagues[25] found that MI in military dental clinics was effective for reducing smokeless tobacco use. The efficacy of MI for smoking cessation has been addressed to a considerable extent in the general medical literature,[26–30] which may explain why the second European Workshop on Tobacco Use Prevention and Cessation for Oral Health Professionals[31] issued a consensus recommendation for the use of MI by oral health professionals for smoking cessation. Not surprisingly, a few recent studies of the benefits of MI for smoking cessation in medical settings used telephonic[32–34] and Internet-based[35,36] interventions, which suggests that such cost-effective telehealth and Internet-based approaches could potentially be clinically effective and cost-effective in dental settings as well. Routine dental checkups represent a good opportunity to promote smoking prevention as well as to promptly identify potential tobacco use disorder. Dental providers' communication and listening skills play an important role in educating patients on the impact of smoking tobacco in both general and oral health, as well as on the numerous benefits of smoking cessation.

## ILLICIT DRUG USE

Although myriad studies of the efficacy of MI for prevention and reduction of illicit substance abuse have appeared in the literature over the past quarter century, the dearth of such in the oral health literature serves to limit conclusions that can be drawn with complete confidence. This limitation is consistent with a 2016 evidence synthesis of MI in general dental practice,[2] in which the investigators noted that although 20,000 articles on MI had been published since 1983, randomized controlled trials accounted for only 200 of these. Their inclusion criteria yielded only 52 studies of MI that could be applied to general dental practice, only 8 of which were of sufficient quality for inclusion in their systematic review. None of the 52 studies addressed illicit substance abuse. Accordingly, dentists interested in MI approaches will be required to extrapolate from the general medical, psychiatric, and substance abuse literature. Over the years, MI approaches have been effective in reducing the use of various types of drugs, including illicit, nonprescription opioids,[37] marijuana,[38] cocaine,[39] and methamphetamine.[40] Although approximately 6% of the population in the United States have an addiction,[41] a review of the literature indicates no current data on the incidence of illegal substance use in dental practice; irrespective, it can be surmised that it is common. Thus, clinicians' abilities to effectively use MI techniques over the course of their relationships will potentially benefit certain patients (particularly those that have not yet developed a severe substance use disorder) without threatening the sanctity of their patient-provider relationships.[42]

By a wide margin, cannabis remains the most abused illicit drug worldwide.[43] In addition to myriad of health concerns associated with its use as levels of delta-9 tetra-hydrocannabinol (THC) increase,[44] there are concerns regarding cannabis use that are unique to dentistry. Many of these concerns pertain to smoking, which remains the most common form of introducing the drug to people's systems.[45] In dental medicine, primary concerns associated with cannabis use include dry mouth and poor oral hygiene in cannabis users contributing to caries,[46] soft tissue diseases (eg, gingival enlargement, thought to relate to the high combustion temperature of cannabis compared with tobacco),[47] fungal infections such as oral candidiasis,[48] and oral cancers.[49] Cocaine and crack use have also been linked to dental problems, including periodontitis,[50] oral mucosal lesions,[51] and palatal perforation.[52] Methamphetamine may be the substance of abuse that has gained the most notoriety over the past 2 decades, with the destruction caused by the habit causing an oral condition known as "meth mouth". In a clinical dental hygiene appointment, generalize, dark, heavy staining associated with methamphetamine use were associated with more severe and frequent caries[53,54] and poor oral hygiene during periods of extended use. Subsequent literature has associated its abuse with xerostomia,[55] bruxism,[56] dental necrosis specifically at the roots of the anterior maxillary teeth,[57] oral cancers,[58] and pain (more than half of methamphetamine users in a recent study[59] reported painful aching in their mouths, discomfort in eating, and consequent avoidance of certain foods). Complicating care are the financial difficulties of chronic methamphetamine abusers, which often leaves extraction of affected teeth as the only dental option.[60] Because of the loss of teeth, a 2010 study[61] found that, despite their relative youth (36.5 years of age), 60% of habitual methamphetamine users were missing a mean of 4.58 teeth (excluding third molars), with 13.3% of the sample already wearing dentures. As a result of dental issues, 28.6% of these patients expressed concern with their dental appearance. The dental hygiene process of care includes a full mouth evaluation. Part of the evaluation involves the use of MI to gain knowledge on frequency of dental visits, health history, and chief concerns. Severe discoloration accompanied by a dry mouth warrants more information on diet, water consumption, and tobacco use, which is used as a gateway question into recreational drug use.

Although numerous studies of the efficacy of MI for reducing and eliminating methamphetamine use appear in the general literature, no such empirical investigations have been published specific to dental medicine. Once again, extrapolation from these studies seems reasonable. A 2015 study noted, "In addition to using dental treatment to improve morale and self-esteem, the concerns about appearance could be used as the basis for brief behavioral interventions in dental settings."[62(p883)] Based on its track record in the treatment of substance abuse disorders, MI in the dental setting can be considered a brief behavioral intervention of choice among this patient population.

## OPIOID USE

Working toward safer and more effective opioid prescribing is another aspect of dental practice in which additional work is imperative. Dentists were indicted during the prescription opioid crisis in the United States for overprescribing during the height of the crisis. For example, in 2011, they were responsible for the prescription of 12% of all immediate-release opioids in the United States, with family practitioners identified as the only group prescribing more.[63] However, to their credit, dentists' decrease in prescribing between 2007 and 2012 was exceeded only by that of emergency department physicians.[64] Irrespective, many believe that dental prescribing rates in general are still too high.[65] Numerous efforts continue to be made to reduce opioid prescribing in dentistry. However, there is little current literature on dealing with individual cases of opioid aberrancy in oral health settings.

As in medicine, improving opioid adherence in dental medicine is crucial in order to make practice safer. In medical settings, MI has been found to be a useful tool to improve medication adherence. For example, a 2014 review[66] of studies of interventions combining cognitive behavior therapy and MI yielded a conclusion of efficacy regarding medication adherence, generally, with a more recent study of older adults with chronic pain at risk for opioid misuse[67] determining that MI increased opioid adherence more specifically. MI has also been found to be a useful tool for enhancing outcomes of opioid tapering.[68] However, in dentistry, there is a complete absence of empirical literature addressing the issue of opioid adherence, with only minimal investigation of medication adherence in general.[69] Accordingly, dentists interested in applying MI with regard to opioid adherence will need to extrapolate from data from studies of such an approach in nondental medicine (discussed earlier) if they are invested in improving adherence and thus the safety of their practice patterns.

To consider MI in dental medicine as a tool to increase opioid adherence, it is important to consider conditions that result in chronic pain. Considerable progress has been made over the past decade to reduce opioid prescribing for acute pain, with an emphasis on consideration of nonopioid medications,[70] wider use of prescription drug monitoring programs,[71] and prescription of smaller amounts of opioids after minor procedures (eg, third-molar extractions).[72] Although these improvements have been caused largely by raising dentists' awareness and institution of specific opioid prescribing protocols, MI is not necessarily the most effective approach for addressing the expectations of patients who had thought that they would receive high dosages of opioid analgesics to treat postprocedure pain. Much of this expectation likely relates to histories of receiving unnecessarily high and potentially dangerous dosages of opioids postprocedure before the onset of the opioid crisis. However, strategies that have been effective in preventing overprescription of opioids for acute pain in dental medicine do not necessarily translate to conditions that may require longer-term analgesia. Even third-molar extractions, in some patients, can result in pain for lengthier periods. For example, Conrad and colleagues[73] determined that, at 7 days postextraction, as many as 15% of those undergoing third-molar removal rated their pain as severe. However, many legitimate chronic pain conditions are treated in dentistry, often with opioids. In addition, because addiction is now rampant in the United States in general, dentists are going to see patients for whom levels of risk for aberrancy are high.[63] These are the cases for which MI interventions for enhanced medication adherence are likely to be most valuable. For example, data indicate that orofacial pain conditions afflict over a quarter of the population, causing disability and a significant reduction of quality of life.[74] Although it has been posited that patients with chronic orofacial pain requiring opioid analgesia should undergo biobehavioral evaluation,[75] finding mental health clinicians with suitable training and experience is not realistic in many areas.[76] As has been the case in pain medicine (as discussed earlier), MI has the potential to be a powerful clinical strategy for use in dental medicine, and accordingly should be considered appropriate in dental medicine as well.

## SUMMARY

For almost half a century, MI has been used as a clinical strategy in the treatment of numerous conditions, most of which involve a significant degree of self-management. Based on the original work on MI by Miller and Rollnick,[1] it is not surprising that many of these conditions have been various types of substance abuse regarding which patients have been ambivalent about changing their behaviors. In dental medicine, a review of the literature indicates that MI's greatest utility has been in the area of improving general oral hygiene in order to reduce caries and other preventable conditions. Irrespective, the literature has shown effectiveness for reduction of the use of dangerous substances, most notably tobacco. However, there have also been a significant number of studies of MI in dentistry as a tool for reducing alcohol abuse, many of which relate to alcohol-related facial trauma.

That such a minute percentage of the thousands of studies on MI in dental medicine have been randomized controlled trials is troubling, because, although the authors have been compelled to extrapolate from studies of MI in general and addiction medicine, the paucity of robust empirical literature has perhaps had an unfortunate adverse impact on the number of dentists willing to use MI to treat substance abuse in their practices more generally. That dentists need help in improving their evaluation and treatment of substance abuse is demonstrated by a study by Parish and colleagues,[77] in which, although more than three-quarters of dentists reported that they questioned patients about issues of substance abuse, two-thirds of those surveyed considered substance abuse assessment to be outside their professional roles. The irony of this professional ambivalence is not lost in this examination of dentists' use of MI, a strategy that gently exploits patients' own ambivalences regarding behavioral change.

Beyond general oral hygiene and the use of tobacco and alcohol, the extrapolation of data on MI from other areas of medicine in which substance abuse treatment occurs is necessary in order to ascertain a reasonable evidence basis in dentistry. Given the prevalence of addiction in American society and data indicating that oral health is very important to 85% of the population,[78] dentists are among the health care providers that individuals see most regularly, thereby putting them in an excellent position to evaluate and perform brief, effective treatments such as MI for their patients at risk for substance abuse. Furthermore, although most dentists in practice work primarily with acute pain conditions (for which the MI approach has not been determined to be of great efficacy), the incidence of chronic orofacial pain that may require longer-term opioid analgesia suggests that MI should be a useful tool in the treatment of these patients, particularly those at higher risk of opioid aberrancy.

In conclusion, MI has built a strong following, with the body of published literature on the topic already impressive. However, more randomized controlled trials are sorely needed to further bolster the evidence basis, particularly in many areas of dental medicine. It is hoped that this article has familiarized the reader with the great potential benefits of MI as a treatment strategy in areas of dentistry in which substance misuse/abuse is often found, and that more dentists will avail themselves of training in this exciting and rewarding treatment approach.

## ACKNOWLEDGMENTS

This work was funded in part by a grant from the Coverys Community Healthcare Foundation.

## REFERENCES

1. Edelstein BL, Ng MW. Chronic disease management strategies of early childhood caries: support from the medical and dental literature. Pediatr Dent 2015;37(3): 281–7.
2. Kay EJ, Vascott D, Hocking A, et al. Motivational interviewing in general dental practice: a review of the evidence. Br Dent J 2016;221(12):785–91.
3. Naidu R, Nunn J, Irwin JD. The effect of motivational interviewing on oral health-care knowledge, attitudes and behaviour of parents and caregivers of preschool children: an exploratory cluster randomised controlled study. BMC Oral Health 2015;15:101.
4. Albino J, Tiwari T. Preventing childhood caries: a review of recent behavioral research. J Dent Res 2016;95(1):35–42.
5. Hinz JG. Teaching dental students motivational interviewing techniques: analysis of a third-year class assignment. J Dent Educ 2010;74(12):1351–6.
6. Arnett M, Korte D, Richards PS, et al. Effect of faculty development activities on dental hygiene faculty perceptions of and teaching about motivational interviewing: a pilot study. J Dent Educ 2017;81(8):969–77.
7. Faustino-Silva DD, Meyer E, Hugo FN, et al. Effectiveness of motivational interviewing training for primary care dentists and dental health technicians: results from a community clinical trial. J Dent Educ 2019;83(5):585–94.
8. Smith AJ, Shepherd JP, Hodgson RJ. Brief interventions for patients with alcohol-related trauma. Br J Oral Maxillofac Surg 1998;36(6):408–15.
9. Goodall CA, Ayoub AF, Crawford A, et al. Nurse delivered brief interventions for hazardous drinkers with alcohol-related facial trauma: a prospective randomized controlled trial. Br J Oral Maxillofac Surg 2008;46:96–101.
10. Lee KH, Hughes A. Would brief alcohol intervention be helpful in facial trauma patients? A narrative review. Oral Maxillofac Surg 2017;21(3):281–8.
11. Miller PM, Ravenel MC, Shealy AE, et al. Alcohol screening in dental patients: the prevalence of hazardous drinking and patients' attitudes about screening and advice. J Am Dent Assoc 2006;137(12):1692–8.
12. Handmaker NS, Miller WR, Manicke M. Findings of a pilot study of motivational interviewing with pregnant drinkers. J Stud Alcohol 1999;60(2):285–7.
13. Monti PM, Barnett NP, Colby SM, et al. Motivational interviewing versus feedback only in emergency care for young adult problem drinking. Addiction 2007;102(8): 1234–43.
14. Gilder DA, Luna JA, Calac D, et al. Acceptability of the use of motivational interviewing to reduce underage drinking in a Native American community. Subst Use Misuse 2011;46(6):836–42.
15. Wiprovnick AE, Kuerbis AN, Morgenstern J. The effects of therapeutic bond within a brief intervention for alcohol moderation for problem drinkers. Psychol Addict Behav 2015;29(1):129–35.
16. Polcin D, Korcha RA, Pugh S, et al. Intensive motivational interviewing for heavy drinking among women. Addict Disord Their Treat 2019;18(2):70–80.
17. McRee B. Open wide! Dental settings are an untapped resource for substance misuse screening and brief intervention. Addiction 2012;107(7):1197–8.

18. Neff JA, Gunsolley JC, Alshatrat SM. Topical trends in tobacco and alcohol articles published in three dental journals, 1980-2010. J Dent Educ 2015;79(6): 671–9.
19. Friedlander AH, Marder SR, Pisegna JR, et al. Alcohol abuse and dependence: psychopathology, medical management and dental implications. J Am Dent Assoc 2003;134(6):731–40.
20. Cruz GD, Ostroff JS, Kumar JV, et al. Preventing and detecting oral cancer. Oral health care providers' readiness to provide health behavior counseling and oral cancer examinations. J Am Dent Assoc 2005;136(5):594–601.
21. Neff JA, Kelley ML, Walters ST, et al. Effectiveness of a Screening and Brief Intervention protocol for heavy drinkers in dental practice: A cluster-randomized trial. J Health Psychol 2015;20(12):1534–48.
22. Koerber A, Crawford J, O'Connell K. The effects of teaching dental students brief motivational interviewing for smoking-cessation counseling: a pilot study. J Dent Educ 2003;67(4):439–47.
23. Rosseel JP, Jacobs JE, Hilberink SR, et al. Experienced barriers and facilitators for integrating smoking cessation advice and support into daily dental practice. A short report. Br Dent J 2011;210(7):E10.
24. Lando HA, Hennrikus D, Boyle R, et al. Promoting tobacco abstinence among older adolescents in dental clinics. J Smok Cessat 2007;2(1):23–30.
25. Severson HH, Peterson AL, Andrews JA, et al. Smokeless tobacco cessation in military personnel: a randomized controlled trial. Nicotine Tob Res 2009;11(6): 73073–8.
26. Litt J. How to provide effective smoking cessation advice in less than a minute without offending the patient. Aust Fam Physician 2002;31(12):1087–94.
27. Soria R, Legido A, Escolano C, et al. A randomised controlled trial of motivational interviewing for smoking cessation. Br J Gen Pract 2006;56(531):768–74.
28. Bock BC, Becker BM, Niaura RS, et al. Smoking cessation among patients in an emergency chest pain observation unit: outcomes of the Chest Pain Smoking Study (CPSS). Nicotine Tob Res 2008;10(10):1523–31.
29. Lim G, Park I, Park S, et al. Effectiveness of smoking cessation using motivational interviewing in patients consulting a pulmonologist. Tuberc Respir Dis (Seoul) 2014;76(6):276–83.
30. Auer R, Gencer B, Tango R, et al. Uptake and efficacy of a systematic intensive smoking cessation intervention using motivational interviewing for smokers hospitalised for an acute coronary syndrome: a multicentre before-after study with parallel group comparisons. BMJ Open 2016;6(9):e011520.
31. Ramseier CA, Warnakulasuriya S, Needleman IG, et al. Consensus report: 2nd European Workshop on tobacco use prevention and cessation for oral health professionals. Int Dent J 2010;60(1):3–6.
32. Taylor KL, Hagerman CJ, Luta G, et al. Preliminary evaluation of a telephone-based smoking cessation intervention in the lung cancer screening setting: A randomized clinical trial. Lung Cancer 2017;108:242–6.
33. Peterson J, Battaglia C, Fehling KB, et al. Perspectives on a home telehealth care management program for veterans with posttraumatic stress disorder who smoke. J Addict Nurs 2017;28(3):117–23.
34. Rogers ES, Fu SS, Krebs P, et al. Proactive tobacco treatment for smokers using Veterans Administration mental health clinics. Am J Prev Med 2018;54(5):620–9.
35. Bommelé J, Schoenmakers TM, Kleinjan M, et al. Targeting hardcore smokers: the effects of an online tailored intervention, based on motivational interviewing techniques. Br J Health Psychol 2017;22(3):644–60.

36. Vogel EA, Belohlavek A, Prochaska JJ, et al. Development and acceptability testing of a Facebook smoking cessation intervention for sexual and gender minority young adults. Internet Interv 2019;15:87–92.

37. Saunders B, Wilkinson C, Phillips M. The impact of a brief motivational intervention with opiate users attending a methadone programme. Addiction 1995;90(3):415–24.

38. Stephens RS, Roffman RA, Curtin L. Comparison of extended versus brief treatments for marijuana use. J Consult Clin Psychol 2000;68(5):898–908.

39. Stotts AL, Schmitz JM, Rhoades HM, et al. Motivational interviewing with cocaine-dependent patients: a pilot study. J Consult Clin Psychol 2001;69(5):858–62.

40. Polcin DL, Bond J, Korcha R, et al. Randomized trial of intensive motivational interviewing for methamphetamine dependence. J Addict Dis 2014;33(3):253–65.

41. Substance Abuse and Mental Health Services Administration. Key substance use and mental health indicators in the United States: results from the 2017 National Survey on Drug Use and Health. 2018. Available at: https://www.google.com/search?q=Substance+Abuse+and+Mental+Health+Services+Administration.+(2018).+Key+Substance+Use+and+Mental+Health+Indicators+in+the+United+States%3A+Results+from+the+2017+National+Survey+on+Drug+Use+and+Health.&rlz=1C1SQJL_enUS797US797&oq=Substance+Abuse+and+Mental+Health+Services+Administration.+(2018).+Key+Substance+Use+and+Mental+Health+Indicators+in+the+United+States%3A+Results+from+the+2017+National+Survey+on+Drug+Use+and+Health.&aqs=chrome..69i57.4665j0j4&sourceid=chrome&ie=UTF-8. Accessed June 27, 2019.

42. Gillam DG, Yusuf H. Brief motivational interviewing in dental practice. Dent J (Basel) 2019;7(2):E51.

43. Global Drug Survey. GDSG2019 key findings report. Available at: https://www.globaldrugsurvey.com/wp-content/themes/globaldrugsurvey/results/GDS2019-Exec-Summary.pdf. Accessed July 1, 2019.

44. Fischer B, Russell C, Sabioni P, et al. Lower-risk cannabis use guidelines: a comprehensive update of evidence and recommendations. Am J Public Health 2017;107(8):e1–12.

45. Russell C, Rueda S, Room R, et al. Routes of administration for cannabis use - basic prevalence and related health outcomes: a scoping review and synthesis. Int J Drug Policy 2018;52:87–96.

46. Schulz-Katterbach MS, Imfeld T, Imfeld C. Cannabis and caries – does regular cannabis use increase the risk of caries in cigarette smokers? Schweiz Monatsschr Zahnmed 2009;119:576–83.

47. Darling MR, Arendorf TM. Effects of cannabis smoking on oral soft tissues. Community Dent Oral Epidemiol 1993;21:78–81.

48. Darling MR, Arendorf TM, Coldrey NA. Effects of cannabis use on oral candidal carriage. J Oral Pathol Med 1990;19:319–21.

49. Zhang ZF, Morgenstern H, Spitz M, et al. Marijuana use and increased risk of squamous cell carcinoma of the head and neck. Cancer Epidemiol Biomarkers Prev 1999;8:1071–8.

50. Antoniazzi R, Zanatta FB, Rösing CK, et al. Association among periodontitis and the use of crack cocaine and other illicit drugs. J Periodontol 2016;87(12):1396–405.

51. Cury PR, Araujo S2, das Graças Alonso Oliveira M, et al. Association between oral mucosal lesions and crack and cocaine addiction in men: a cross-sectional study. Environ Sci Pollut Res Int 2018;25(20):19801–7.

52. Brand H1, Gonggrijp S, Blanksma CJ. Cocaine and oral health. Br Dent J 2008; 204(7):365–9.
53. Venker D. Crystal methamphetamine and the dental patient. Iowa Dent J 1999; 85(4):34.
54. Shaner JW. Caries associated with methamphetamine abuse. J Mich Dent Assoc 2002;84(9):42–7.
55. Saini T, Edwards PC, Kimmes NS, et al. Etiology of xerostomia and dental caries among methamphetamine abusers. Oral Health Prev Dent 2005;3(3):189–95.
56. Curtis EK. Meth mouth: a review of methamphetamine abuse and its oral manifestations. Gen Dent 2006;54(2):125–9.
57. Richards JR, Brofeldt BT. Patterns of tooth wear associated with methamphetamine use. J Periodontol 2000;71:1371–4.
58. Smart RJ, Rosenberg M. Methamphetamine abuse: medical and dental considerations. J Mass Dent Soc 2005;54(2):44–6, 48-49.
59. Mukherjee A, Dye BA, Clague J, et al. Methamphetamine use and oral health-related quality of life. Qual Life Res 2018;27(12):3179–90.
60. Williams N, Covington JS 3rd. Methamphetamine and meth mouth: an overview. J Tenn Dent Assoc 2006;86:32–5.
61. Shetty V, Mooney LJ, Zigler CM, et al. The relationship between methamphetamine use and increased dental disease. J Am Dent Assoc 2010;141(3):307–18.
62. Shetty V, Harrell L, Murphy DA, et al. Dental disease patterns in methamphetamine users: Findings in a large urban sample. J Am Dent Assoc 2015; 146(12):875–85.
63. Denisco RC, Kenna GA, O'Neil MG, et al. Prevention of prescription opioid abuse: the role of the dentist. J Am Dent Assoc 2011;142(7):800–10.
64. Levy B, Paulozzi L, Mack KA, et al. Trends in opioid analgesic-prescribing rates by specialty, U.S., 2007-2012. Am J Prev Med 2015;49(3):409–13.
65. Suda KJ, Durkin MJ, Calip GS, et al. Comparison of opioid prescribing by dentists in the United States and England. JAMA Netw Open 2019;2(5):e194303.
66. Spoelstra SL, Schueller M, Hilton M, et al. Interventions combining motivational interviewing and cognitive behaviour to promote medication adherence: a literature review. J Clin Nurs 2014;24:1163–73.
67. Chang YP, Compton P, Almeter P, et al. The effect of motivational interviewing on prescription opioid adherence among older adults with chronic pain. Perspect Psychiatr Care 2015;51:211–2119.
68. Sullivan MD, Turner JA, DiLodovico C, et al. Prescription opioid taper support for outpatients with chronic pain: a randomized controlled trial. J Pain 2017;18(3): 308–18.
69. Hersh EV, Ciancio SG, Kuperstein AS, et al. An evaluation of 10 percent and 20 percent benzocaine gels in patients with acute toothaches: efficacy, tolerability and compliance with label dose administration directions. J Am Dent Assoc 2013;144(5):517–26.
70. Wong YJ, Keenan J, Hudson K, et al. Opioid, NSAID, and OTC analgesic medications for dental procedures: PEARL Network findings. Compend Contin Educ Dent 2016;37(10):710–8.
71. McCauley JL, Gilbert GH, Cochran DL, et al. Prescription drug monitoring program use: National Dental PBRN results. JDR Clin Trans Res 2019;4(2):178–86.
72. Tompach PC, Wagner CL, Sunstrum AB, et al. Investigation of an opioid prescribing protocol after third molar extraction procedures. J Oral Maxillofac Surg 2019; 77(4):705–14.

73. Conrad SM, Blakey GH, Shugars DA, et al. Patients' perception of recovery after third molar surgery. J Oral Maxillofac Surg 1999;57(11):1288–94.

74. Shueb SS, Nixdorf DR, John MT, et al. What is the impact of acute and chronic orofacial pain on quality of life? J Dent 2015;43:1203–10.

75. Burgess JA. Orofacial pain: what to look for, how to treat, part 1. Consultant 2006; 46(1):25.

76. Darnall BD, Carr DB, Schatman ME. Pain psychology and the biopsychosocial model of pain treatment: ethical imperatives and social responsibility. Pain Med 2017;18:1413–5.

77. Parish CL, Pereyra MR, Pollack HA, et al. Screening for substance misuse in the dental care setting: findings from a nationally representative survey of dentists. Addiction 2015;110(9):1516–23.

78. American Dental Association. Survey: more Americans want to visit the dentist. ADA News; 2018. Available at: https://www.ada.org/en/publications/ada-news/2018-archive/march/survey-more-americans-want-to-visit-the-dentist. Accessed July 9, 2019.

# Interprofessional Collaboration in the Assessment and Management of Substance Use Risk

Ronald J. Kulich, PhD[a,b,c,]*, David A. Keith, BDS, FDSRCS, DMD[d,e],
Alexis A. Vasciannie[f], Huw F. Thomas, BDS, MS, PhD[g]

## KEYWORDS

- Substance use disorder • Dentistry • Barriers • Opioids • Risk

## KEY POINTS

- Substance use disorder assessment strategies are increasingly being employed by dentistry, while adequate evaluation requires reaching out to other cotreating providers and collaborating on patient care.
- The field of dentistry has a range of barriers often not experienced in other professions, including limitations on e-record communication and clinical practice setting often isolated from the patient's general medical care.
- Barriers can be overcome if the dentist facilitates communication.

The problem of controlled substance risk assessment and management is well known. Dentists have been increasingly identified as health care practitioners who can be on the front line to identify individuals at risk, effectively managing their dental care and providing appropriate triage to other health care colleagues who can deliver additional evaluation and management of their potential substance use disorders. In a systematic review, Badri and colleagues[1] identified collaboration between health care professionals and dentistry to be a major barrier to adherence for pediatric patients, a

[a] Tufts University School of Dental Medicine, Department of Diagnostic Sciences, Craniofacial Pain & Headache Center, 1 Kneeland Street, Boston, MA 02111, USA; [b] Department of Anesthesia, Critical Care and Pain Medicine, Massachusetts General Hospital, Boston, MA, USA; [c] Department of Psychiatry, Massachusetts General Hospital, Boston, MA, USA; [d] Massachusetts General Hospital, 55 Fruit Street, Boston, MA 02114, USA; [e] Oral and Maxillofacial Surgery, Harvard School of Dental Medicine, Boston, MA, USA; [f] Department of Diagnostic Sciences, Tufts University School of Dental Medicine, 1 Kneeland Street, Boston, MA 02111, USA; [g] Tufts University School of Dental Medicine, One Kneeland Street, Room 1163, Boston, MA 02111, USA
* Corresponding author. Tufts University School of Dental Medicine, Craniofacial Pain & Headache Center, 1 Kneeland Street, Boston, MA 02111.
E-mail address: RKULICH@mgh.harvard.edu

Dent Clin N Am 64 (2020) 571–583
https://doi.org/10.1016/j.cden.2020.02.006
0011-8532/20/© 2020 Elsevier Inc. All rights reserved.

population where the importance of working across disciplines would appear most obvious. Although there is some debate for expanding dentistry's scope of practice, few argue that increased collaboration between dentistry and other health care professions benefits the patient and the profession.

Notwithstanding a national push to promote interprofessional education and multidisciplinary clinical care, dentistry continues to lag behind other health care professions in addressing this issue. As management of patients with complex medical conditions has required more robust medical knowledge, other disciplines have moved forward with interprofessional collaboration by establishing teams to evaluate and care for patients, integrate e-medical records, and work to.

Part of the problem may stem from current dental school training. In a review encouraging interprofessional collaborative practice, Cole and colleagues[2] explain that "interprofessional education occurs when two or more professions learn about, from, and with each other to enable effective collaboration and improve health outcomes." Although dental schools adhere to this definition, they tend to provide interprofessional education by offering lectures that cross dental disciplines, providing parallel educational efforts with medical schools, or adding a series of didactic lectures taught by basic scientists or mental health professionals. Few health professions schools promote care in which the dentist functions as an active member of the health care team, a concept that is critical in assessing patients with substance use risk. A recent American Dental Education Association publication asserts that a broader perspective should be considered, noting that "dentistry will and should become more closely integrated with medicine and the health care system on all levels: research, education, and patient care."[3] Similarly, in a response to the Miller and colleagues[4] commentary on the question as to whether dentistry has a role in health care, Keith and Kulich suggest that this effort needs to be at the predoctoral training level on substance use risk, involving "collaboration on complex cases where each discipline can provide critical input within their expertise. For example, we are now fortunate to have joint programs in Massachusetts where dental, medical, pharmacy and nursing students review complex cases and receive education on opioid overdose reversal with naloxone as part of this training."[5] As part of this effort, Patterson and associates[6] integrated dental (n = 74), medical (n = 205), and pharmacy (n = 300) students for a series of half-day programs. Faculty from each discipline developed an integrated teaching case using an acute orofacial pain patient presenting to the emergency department, concurrently on assisted suboxone treatment for opioid use disorder. Students worked collaboratively to address effective pain management for the simulated patient, develop risk mitigation strategies, and interpret the results from the state Prescription Drug Monitoring Program (PDMP). Issues of opioid adverse effects and risk for overdose were addressed, with pharmacists in training demonstrating how to administer various formulations of naloxone. Although more than half of medical and pharmacy students had exposure to naloxone administration prior to the training, fewer than 10% of dentists in training had similar exposure. Results showed that 70% of dental students now felt that they would take necessary action to intervene with an opioid overdose, and the majority identified the correct interval for second-dose administration.[6]

Aside from the cross-disciplinary knowledge acquired by the dental student, programs such as this can promote a level of comfort around the delivery of collaborative care. Medical fields such as oncology and pediatrics already are familiar with cointerviewing patients. This approach may reduce patient burden as identical sensitive questions many not need to be repeated, and patient comfort may be enhanced with increased cross-communication and consistent patient messaging. Similarly, Tufts Orofacial Pain Center, a university-based clinic, conducts assessments in this manner for its most complex patients, many of whom present with substance use risk. For complex patients who present with polypharmacy, they concurrently interview the patient with the dentist, neurologist, and pain psychologist. In the absence of a fully integrated dental practice within a comprehensive health care setting, these efforts are unlikely to be implemented within general dentistry practices. Nonetheless, data from other medical fields provide support for cost-effectiveness, reduced discharge rates, and enhanced patient adherence.[7,8]

## COMMUNICATION AND COLLABORATING WITH COTREATING CLINICIANS

Integrating health care disciplines into the patient's overall care has received understandable resistance, even for very complex patients. Because the general dentist is not typically integrated into the medical decision-making teams, identifying responsible medical and addiction psychiatry sources can be an even greater challenge, which is especially alarming when the patient may be at-risk for overdose.

As early as the 1990s, the field of pain medicine came under scrutiny for abuses of interdisciplinary treatment, where there often was a failure to adequately screen patients who might require such intensive care. At the time, a medical director of a large health maintenance organization opined that some interdisciplinary pain centers "never saw a discipline they didn't like."[9] As a result of billing abuses and resistance from insurance carriers, many interdisciplinary pain centers went out of business. In response, the American Pain Society commissioned a managed care committee to address the issue and efforts were made to accommodate concerns of third party payors.[9] A similar process is currently underway with respect to interdisciplinary addiction medicine facilities where examples of fraud are now surfacing.[10] For example, interdisciplinary addiction programs now offer equine therapy, with many of these integrated services being marketed in the absence of supporting research. Even in the best scenario where the dentist identifies an at-risk patient abusing a substance, where does one responsibly go to refer and collaborate?

Some dentists have already identified and established relationships with local mental health and substance abuse treatment providers, usually pre-empting the need for finding other resources. Ideally, many at-risk patients will also arrive at the dental practice with their cotreating clinician already in place, most likely a primary care physician (PCP) or substance use disorder specialist. Substance use clinicians can have backgrounds in internal medicine with specialty board certification in addiction medicine. Similarly, some psychiatrists can have added board certification in addiction psychiatry. Many patients are treated by doctoral level clinical psychologists specializing in addiction disorders, as well as social workers and licensed chemical dependency counselors. Emergency evaluation and inpatient treatment services should be readily accessible as resources for anyone undergoing formal substance abuse treatment. Although many of these services are valuable adjuncts to effective substance use disorder care, group support services such as Alcoholics Anonymous are not considered treatment providers. Support group programs should not be considered an adequate or exclusive referral option for care. Unfortunately, as responsible community or state-based services become increasingly identified, dental practices are typically not on regional state notification lists. For example, information about naloxone distribution is more commonly provided to medical providers, and many states offer distribution without prescriptions at various sites. The dentist will need to be proactive in identifying relevant local resources and urge state dental societies to better inform their members about substance use disorder care. Recently Massachusetts PDMP has added a list of resources that is imbedded in each patient's database.[11]

Utilizing government- and nonprofit-based rapid access referral services can be an effective option. Details on formal outpatient and inpatient local facilities can be accessed on the Substance Abuse and Mental Health Services Administration Web site.[12] The National SAMHSA Helpline is free, confidential, and available around the clock as a referral and information resource. Dentists can reach out to this resource for referral purposes, as well as individuals and families with mental and/or substance use disorders. Structured controlled substance risk screeners such as the NIDA Quick Screen also link dentists to specific resources for patients.[13]

## SMOKING CESSATION SUPPORTED BY DENTISTRY

Dentists have been on the forefront of care with nicotine abuse, with the effects of vaping now being addressed by national and regional dental societies.[14] The American Dental Association (2019) clearly notes that "because of the oral health implications of tobacco use, dental practices may provide a uniquely effective setting for tobacco use recognition, prevention, and cessation; dental professionals can help smokers quit by consistently identifying patients who smoke, advising them to quit, and offering them information about cessation treatment."[15] Although dentists may be qualified to counsel the patient, make the referral, and prescribe smoking cessation medications,[16] few follow this approach, despite data showing its cost efficiency.[17] Agaku and colleagues[18] found that 31% of dentists advised patients to quit smoking, in contrast to 65% of physicians. Only 24.5% of dentists went beyond the simple advice to quit. Further complicating the situation for patients who are concurrently using regularly prescribed opioids, comorbid use of tobacco or cannabis significantly increased the likelihood of the patient being nonadherent or showing some drug aberrancy.[19,20] Even in cases where the dentist choses to defer prescribing appropriate smoking cessation products, collaborating with the PCP remains a mainstay of good care. Smoking, vaping, and/or excessive cannabis use all can negatively impact the oral cavity. Additionally, use of these substances can also predict the presence of other comorbid substance use disorders and should be considered a risk factor suggesting that a more comprehensive controlled substance risk assessment be conducted. The dentist can then confer and collaborate with appropriate providers who have expertise in substance use disorder treatment.

## ATTITUDES TOWARD SUBSTANCE USE

The stigma associated with substance use disorder is common across all health care provider groups, including dentistry. Dentists also significantly underestimate the prevalence of substance abuse disorders within their patient populations, and the problem is not exclusive to the United States. Priyadarshini and colleagues found that 86.2% of dentists did not believe that substance use disorder was a problem in their practices.[21] Training has been shown to alter these beliefs.[22] Although attitudes can be changed when the dentist institutes standardized controlled substance risk screening in the practice and collaborates with colleagues who regularly evaluate and treat individuals with substance use disorders.

Stigma associated with substance abuse disorder can lead to denial, reduced access to and poor quality of care, and nonadherence. Failure to understand substance use disorders and related mental disorders often underpins the problem.[23] Although easier to implement in dental schools, coevaluations can dramatically change the clinician's attitude toward addiction and mental illness. Continuing education programs are attempting to address this issue with patient simulations, an effort that better promotes understanding and empathy. Dentists and most health care providers also lack an understanding that substance use disorders, by their nature, are reoccurring illnesses, and relapses are common. As with other addictive disorders such as smoking, few remain abstinent after the first attempt. That being said, treatment has been shown to be effective. Patients most benefit when support is made available through the family, employer, and health care providers. An example of this more enlightened approach closer to home is the issue of dental colleagues who may suffer from substance use disorder. Five percent to 10% of dentists experience a drug or alcohol problem during their careers.[24] Once addiction takes over, they become too ashamed to seek help for fear of public exposure and reprisal by the licensing board. Most states support dentists through a confidential diversion program, creating an incentive to seek help. As a result, dentists get the help they need, and patients get the protection they deserve. Dentists who complete a diversion program recover at a rate of 80% to 90% - 3 times that of the general public. Massachusetts is currently developing a similar program. An Act Establishing a Dentist Diversion Program (H.238) is now being considered.[25]

## DISCLOSURE TO THE PATIENT

In the complex situation where substance use risk is present, a frank discussion with the patient is always prudent. When a patient presents with high risk of controlled substance misuse, and dental care is planned, a supportive explanation about the need to communicate with other prescribing clinicians is necessary. Normalizing the conversation is the first step, indicating that the patient's safety is ensured and arriving at the best plan for providing effective pain relief if a procedure is planned. Although it is always ideal to seek consent from the patient, there are no HIPAA (Health Insurance Portability and Accountability Act) barriers for communication between providers, even where substance misuse or abuse is discussed. Reviewing PDMP results with the patient also is advisable, especially in cases where the results are consistent with the patient's self-report. Finally, documenting the patient's response to the plan is necessary, and exact quotes from the patient should be placed in the record. This process is an integral part of the verbal informed consent, and a positive step toward collaborating with the patient on his or her care. There are cases where the patient may adamantly decline to have the dentist contact the cotreating physician or other dental providers, as in the case of William M (**Box 1**). Although discussion of the patient's rationale for restricted communication can be helpful, this is typically a flag for other risk factors of possible substance abuse or diversion. Although the patient may require dental care, the dentist is typically not obligated to undertake treatment with such unreasonable restrictions in place.

## FAMILY, CAREGIVERS, AND SIGNIFICANT OTHERS

The role for a caregiver is well established in children and adolescents, as well as cases where the patient has impaired cognitive status or may not be competent to handle medical decision making around his or her care. In residential treatment programs for substance use disorder, there is a 9.62% increased program completion rate when family members are actively involved.[26] Involving the family in assessment and care is a well-established component of alcohol use disorder treatment, and similar data have emerged with opioid use disorder.[27] Family involvement also results in better outcome with smoking cessation.[28] In framing the communication, it is reasonable to suggest that the spouse caregiver join in the assessment, and the authors typically use the comment that "your spouse knows you better than anyone else, and her/his input will be valuable

**Box 1**
**Interaction with a high-risk patient**

D: Hi Mr. Morton. We're still working on a plan, but we need to talk some more. We want to help make this go as smooth as possible for you so that your procedure goes well. I know that you've been in a lot of pain lately. We checked your medication history through our prescription drug monitoring program, and it looks like you're also under treatment with some other doctors. We're required to check before prescribing certain pain medications. The record shows you've been on a lot of pain medications that we didn't have listed on the medical history. It looks like you've also been on a number of medications for anxiety and maybe a muscle relaxant.

W: I have a lot of pain, and I know my teeth are really bad. I just can't get somebody to help me. I'm desperate, and I've been trying everything I can. Most of the other medications are not related to my teeth; they're for my back and neck pain. This is a state-run database? What right do they have to get this information? I'll sue them and you; it's preposterous and unfair. All I want is to get rid of my pain!

D: I'm sorry to hear that. I'm happy to go through the prescription record with you to see if there are any inaccuracies. I see you saw Dr. Smith recently (review PDMP summary with patient).

W: Yes, he fixed my ankle last winter.

D: You have also seen Dr. Brown?

W: Yes, I went to him for this tooth, but he wouldn't do anything to help me.

D: And Dr. Jones?

W: He was at that urgent care clinic in town. I sprained my back.

D: Okay, you've been seeing a number of other doctors recently, and each are prescribing for you. Since you're taking a number of medications from a lot of doctors, and we also know you're drinking quite a bit from what you told us, this can impact your safety if we're considering other medications through our practice.

D: Are you seeing any counsellors or mental health providers?

W: Yeah, I am working with someone, I have a primary care doctor, but what does that have to do with getting my teeth fixed?

D: We can't treat you safely unless all of the doctors are communicating about your medical care. Your dental care also will have a better outcome if you are seeing your counselor regularly and following instructions from your primary physician. Before prescribing any controlled substances, I'd first like to have a discussion with your primary physician or the other doctor who is primarily following you for pain, anxiety, or substance use. Also, with respect to your upcoming dental procedure, we generally can manage a problem like this with lower-risk medications, and you'll still get very good pain relief. We won't be writing opioids for your care today, but I'm happy to call your primary doctor and discuss the plan for pain management.

W: OK, I really need this work done on my teeth. I don't want you calling anybody though. It's none of your business; you don't have permission to do that.

D: It's entirely up to you Mr. Morton, but we can't care for you with those restrictions. We can discuss other emergency referral options, but you do need to follow-up and get proper dental care for these problems.

in coming up with the best treatment plan." The family member may be able to better recall the patient's medication regimen or past treatments, and also may elect to comment on the patient concerns or any issues of adherence. In matters where sensitive subject matter is discussed, a notation can be placed in the record indicating that the patient gave permission for the spouse to participate. Particularly in the case of substance use disorder risk assessment, alliance with the spouse will predict a better outcome, and further reduce the dentist's role in caring for the whole patient. Exceptions include situations where domestic violence may be suspected, an area of assessment that also should be included in every initial comprehensive dental and medical history. There are cases where the spouse or caregiver is promoting or enabling substance use disorder behaviors, and there also exist pediatric and gerontology cases where parents or care givers have used dental and medical visits to acquire and divert controlled substances. Thorough assessment of the patient is always warranted, with extra caution where risks are present.

Finally, caretakers and family should not be employed as health care translators in dental or medical settings. While in-person medical translation may not always be possible in many dental practice, other phone services are available to responsibly address the issues. Independent of language barriers, cultural issues also come into play when assessing the patient at-risk for substance use disorder.[29]

## INITIATING THE COMMUNICATION WITH PRIMARY CARE OR ADDICTION MEDICINE

Communication with other relevant treatment clinicians is a mainstay of care for the complex patient who presents with substance abuse or misuse risk. Whether it is the high-risk patient attempting to doctor shop for hydrocodone or a more straightforward patient being referred for smoking cessation, some personal contact with the other provider increases the likelihood of an improved clinical outcome. When time allows, calling the cotreating physician while the patient is in the examination chair provides an ideal scenario. Again, it can be stated that this does not violate HIPPAA regulations.

Although the goals of the call vary, the typical conversation should include the plans for dental care and a discussion of the need for analgesics, patient's medical and/or psychiatric comorbidities, any concerning inconsistencies in the patient's report, and query on other aspects of the patient's medical care that may be relevant. It may be the case where the dentist knows the patient's medical and mental health status much better than the treating physician. Nonetheless, the internist or addiction medicine specialist can likely provide relevant information on medical comorbidities associated with substance use risk, status of the patient's adherence to treatment, or other factors that may directly impact the patients dental care and plans for follow-up. Most importantly, the dentist may have identified substance use risk factors, and providing this information permits the physician to move forward with improved care.

Not all treating physicians are the same with respect to cooperative communication or skill in providing responsible medical care. For example, the dentist may encounter a patient who presents with extremely high-dose opioids where minimal medical monitoring is occurring, and the physician might be unaware of a complex polypharmacy problem that puts the patient at risk. Where there are barriers to communication with the other treating team members, it is fully within the dentist's scope of practice to facilitate a referral for consultation with addiction medicine or psychiatry, refer a patient for substance use disorder consultation, or triage for emergency services where there is an imminent risk to the patient. It is entirely possible that many other prior treating physicians and dentists failed to conduct an adequate substance use assessment and even failed to check the prescription drug monitoring program while concurrently writing high-risk prescriptions. The dentist is in an excellent position to document this risk.

Most cotreating providers will welcome new data that improve patient care, and patients appreciate this extra attention to safety. Although discussions of this type are delicate, disclosing sensitive information has been shown to result in the patient feeling emotionally closer to the clinician. As a result, adherence with treatment recommendations and patient satisfaction may be improved. There is a subset of patients who may push back, and the most difficult scenarios occur with the patient who suffers from active substance use disorder and feels desperate and angry about his or her current status. **Box 1** covers a scenario that occurred with discussion of controlled substance issues. In the scenario the patient required necessary dental work. He previously admitted to drinking large amounts of alcohol and use of illicit substances in the earlier brief screener administered by the dental hygienist. A review of the PDMP revealed that he had obtained 151 prescriptions, 97 prescriptions for opioids, and 20 for benzodiazepines. Several of his prescribers had been dentists, and he had visited multiple pharmacies. He was clearly a high-risk patient, and communication with his PCP was essential. The referral to a mental health or addiction specialist can be made through the patient's PCP or directly. Having these interdisciplinary contacts available is vital for the dentist who treats complex patients, so the referral can be made securely, and the patient feels that continuity of care is being maintained. Suggesting that the patient find a resource with no follow-up from the referring clinician can seem to be a strategy for getting rid of the patient-sometimes called a faux referral. When seeing a complex patient for the first time it is always valuable to mention that care will be provided in an interdisciplinary fashion and that subsequent referrals to other specialists may be anticipated. This avoids the appearance of these referrals being made when all else fails or as a last resort-a scenario that universally leads to frustration, noncompliance, and unnecessary and sometimes harmful treatment.

Although the previously mentioned case may appear to be an extreme example, many such cases get overlooked if the dentist is unaware of the patient's history. Even in the case of active substance abuse, doctor shopping, or possible diversion, the patient still deserves responsible dental care. The dentist can contact the treating physician and offer guidance. In this case, contact with the dentist may be the first step for this patient in addressing his probable active substance use disorder.

## FAMILIARITY AND COMFORT WITH THE BASICS OF RISK ASSESSMENT AND SUBSTANCE USE MANAGEMENT

In order to provide the best care and encourage effective communication across other health care providers, dentists are encouraged to familiarize themselves with the basic substance use disorder risk factors discussed in other articles in this article, as well as access other sources such as the Centers for Disease Control and Prevention (CDC) Guideline for Prescribing Opioids for Chronic Pain.[30] Similarly, the discussion with treating physicians can be more productive when the dentist is familiar with the common controlled substances agents on state prescription drugs monitoring programs. Some state PDMP Web sites offer details on drugs discovered in the patient electronic query, although other sources also are widely available.[31]

The Controlled Substance Risk Mitigation Checklist is discussed elsewhere in more detail. Interprofessional collaboration remains important throughout the components of a good substance use risk assessment (**Fig. 1**). Not all patients require every component of assessment, although it is hoped that this outline provides a framework for comprehensive assessment. Such an assessment is an ongoing process, and substance abuse risk may change over time. The dentist may learn that the patient recently has been started on chronic opioids or benzodiazepines, a change not

| Comprehensive risk assessment | Data from special sources |
|---|---|
| <ul><li>Provide rationale for questions</li><li>Assess pain</li><li>Assess current substance use, including legal and illicit substances</li><li>Assess medical and psychosocial risk factors</li><li>Assess dental risk factors</li><li>Analyze relevant PE and/or MSE findings</li></ul> | <ul><li>Check PDMP and interpret findings</li><li>Complete screening questionnaires (NIDA quick-screen)</li><li>Communicate with other treating clinicians</li><li>Communicate with patient and family members/caregivers</li></ul> |
| **Disposition & follow-up** | **Ongoing collaboration & assessment** |
| <ul><li>Determine/document level of risk prior to prescribing</li><li>Individualized treatment recommendations</li><li>Determine likelihood of adherence/follow-up</li><li>Make appropriate referrals: MH, SA, pain care</li><li>Instruct patient re: safe Rx disposal</li><li>Assess need for continued monitoring and/or higher level of care</li></ul> | <ul><li>Communicate and collaborate with other care providers</li><li>Perform periodic reassessment of pain, SUD risk, and mental health comorbidities</li><li>Attend to special at-risk populations that develop over time: The NAS patient, the patient requiring naloxone, adolescents, etc.</li></ul> |

**Fig. 1.** Controlled substance risk mitigation checklist.

disclosed by the patient. These data may come from communication with the internist or mental health provider or from unexpected PDMP results. Conversely, a reassessment by the dentist may reveal aspects of the patient's current status that are critical to improving care offered by other providers.

## INTERPROFESSIONAL CARE WITHIN THE DENTAL OFFICE: THE ROLE OF THE DENTAL HYGIENIST

The importance of interprofessional care within the dentist's office cannot be understated, and the dental hygienist must be formally integrated into the risk-assessment and management process.[32,33] As underscored in other articles in this series, the dental hygienist is qualified to use standardized risk screeners such as the SBIRT (Screening Brief Intervention and Referral to Treatment)/NIDA (National Institute on Drug Abuse) Quick Screen assessment, and interview the patient on sensitive subject matters.[34] Indeed, the hygienist may know the patient better than the dentist, and thus function as a critical member of the interdisciplinary team. Depending on the state, hygienists also can function as delegates for Prescription Drug Monitoring searches, working under the dentist's license as the controlled substance provider. The hygienist can assist with documentation of risk factors, an activity fully within the scope of their practice.

## ACQUIRING AND SENDING PATIENT NOTES

A scant 5% of dentists regularly request medical notes for patients, and recent data from the authors' group show that the attitude toward acquiring notes is mixed.[35] Even dentists with an expertise in addiction medicine and/or pain may hesitate to seek out medical records. In part, this hesitancy may be due to barriers the dentist has with medical e-records access. There has been an increasing effort to integrate electronic medical records across multiple health care provider groups within each state, although this integration has not extended to most dental practices. Other health care providers can easily view medical records, although dental records are not commonly included in these databases. Similarly, patient portals such as Gateway online records are commonly shared between large medical groups,[36] although they again, typically do not include dental records. Current dental e-record systems are sparse with documentation and assessment of common medical conditions, especially those where mental health or substance abuse patient data are required, further complicating the problem. In contrast, newer medical e-record systems can readily accommodate structured assessment protocols such as the Patient-Reported Outcomes Measurement Information System (PROMIS) measures.[37] The assessments often include mental health and substance use risk. Reviewing records and communicating with e-documentation remain a critical area of development for dentistry, which likely will be better addressed in the future.

## TELEMEDICINE, INTERPROFESSIONAL CARE, AND DENTISTRY

The movement toward telemedicine has focused on addressing barriers with rural or underserved areas. Estai and colleagues[38] outline an interesting application in Australia, highlighting the benefits and various barriers. Issues of billing, documentation, and medico-legal liability require consideration, although the benefits may eventually outweigh any risks. Rather than focusing solely on providing improved dental service to underserved areas, barriers to interdisciplinary assessment and care of the complex patient also may be mitigated with this approach. However, most dentists will likely continue to practice in relatively isolated groups.

## SUMMARY AND FUTURE DIRECTIONS

Interprofessional collaboration has received growing attention in dentistry, and it is especially vital to bring health care professionals together when assessing and managing the patient with substance use risk. Although there are barriers, practicing dentists can improve patient outcomes by reaching out to others who are concurrently managing the complex patient. It is also an opportunity to bring better recognition to the role that dentistry plays in the overall health of the patient. It is surely within the dentist's scope of practice to evaluate and refer the patient with substance use risk and participate in his or her care as an active team member, with the dental hygienist assuming an active role. As a team member, the dentist should actively participate in what is necessarily an ongoing evaluation process for the at-risk patient. As with other dental and medical conditions, the patient's status likely changes over time, and the dentist is well-positioned to offer input on those changes. Standardized risk assessment may help to familiarize the dentist with the risk assessment process and promote comfort with dentistry's expanding role in health care. Technological methods may further ease financial and time burdens and approaches that have already been well-tested in other health care settings. Finally, interdisciplinary care also assumes an increasing role for collaborative input by the patient's family, a resource that predicts to improved success with any substance use disorder approach to care.

## DISCLOSURE

Partial support was received for the preparation of this article through a grant from "The Coverys Community Healthcare Foundation".

## REFERENCES

1. Badri P, Saltaji H, Flores-Mir C, et al. Factors affecting childrens adherence to regular dental attendance. J Am Dent Assoc 2014;145(8):817–28.
2. Cole J, Martin M, Dodge W, et al. Interprofessional collaborative practice: how could dentistry participate? J Dent Educ 2018;82(5):441–5.
3. Palatta A, Cook BJ, Anderson EL, et al. 20 years beyond the crossroads: the path to interprofessional education at U.S. dental schools. J Dent Educ 2015;79(8): 982–96.
4. Miller CS, Rhodus NL, Robinson JC. MyView: does dentistry have a role in health care?. 2018. Available at: https://www.ada.org/en/publications/ada-news/viewpoint/my-view/2018/november/myview-does-dentistry-have-a-role-in-health-care. Accessed December 29, 2019.
5. Hoang E, Keith DA, Kulich R. Controlled substance misuse risk assessment and prescription monitoring database use by dentists. J Am Dent Assoc 2019;150(5): 383–92.
6. Patterson E. Clinical models for risk mitigation in dental medicine. Presented at: Substance Risk Mitigation for Clinicians Conference. Boston, Massachusetts, June 8, 2019.
7. Bell PF, Semelka MW, Bigdeli L. Drug testing incoming residents and medical students in family medicine training: a survey of program policies and practices. J Grad Med Educ 2015;7(1):59–64.
8. Litts JK, Gartner-Schmidt JL, Clary MS, et al. Impact of laryngologist and speech pathologist coassessment on outcomes and billing revenue. Laryngoscope 2015; 125(9):2139–42.
9. Lande S, Kulich RJ, editors. Managed care and pain. Glenview (IL): American Pain Society; 2000.
10. Rothenberg Z. Trends in combating fraud and abuse in substance use disorder treatment. Journal of Health Care Compliance 2018;20(5):13–20.

11. Clinical Services - Opioid Stewardship. VigiLanz. Available at: https://vigilanzcorp. com/opioid-stewardship/. Accessed January 27, 2020.

12. Elliott S. Find treatment. SAMHSA. Available at: https://www.samhsa.gov/find-treatment. Accessed January 26, 2020.

13. NIDA drug screening tool. Available at: https://www.drugabuse.gov/nmassist/. Accessed January 26, 2020.

14. ALHarthi SS, BinShabaib M, Akram Z, et al. Impact of cigarette smoking and vaping on the outcome of full-mouth ultrasonic scaling among patients with gingival inflammation: a prospective study. Clin Oral Investig 2019;23(6):2751–8.

15. Tobacco use and cessation. Available at: https://www.ada.org/en/member-center/oral-health-topics/tobacco-use-and-cessation. Accessed December 30, 2019.

16. Bloom EL, Carpenter MJ, Walaska K, et al. Pilot trial of nicotine replacement therapy sampling in a dental care clinic. J Smok Cessat 2019;1–5. https://doi.org/10. 1017/jsc.2019.17.

17. Csikar JI, Douglas GV, Pavitt S, et al. The cost-effectiveness of smoking cessation services provided by general dental practice, general medical practice, pharmacy and NHS Stop Smoking Services in the North of England. Community Dent Oral Epidemiol 2015;44(2):119–27.

18. Agaku IT, Ayo-Yusuf OA, Vardavas CI. A comparison of cessation counseling received by current smokers at US dentist and physician offices during 2010–2011. Am J Public Health 2014;104(8). https://doi.org/10.2105/ajph.2014.302049.

19. Rajabi A, Dehghani M, Shojaei A, et al. Association between tobacco smoking and opioid use: A meta-analysis. Addict Behav 2019;92:225–35.

20. Dibenedetto DJ, Weed VF, Wawrzyniak KM, et al. The association between cannabis use and aberrant behaviors during chronic opioid therapy for chronic pain. Pain Med 2017;19(10):1997–2008.

21. Priyadarshini S, Sahoo P, Jena D, et al. Knowledge, attitude and practice of dental professionals towards substance use. J Int Soc Prev Community Dent 2019;9(1):65.

22. Calleja NG, Rodems E, Groh CJ, et al. Differences in substance use-related attitudes across behavioral and primary health trainees: a screening, brief intervention, and referral to treatment (SBIRT) training investigation. Alcohol Treat Q 2019; 38(1):106–25.

23. Brondani MA, Alan R, Donnelly L. Stigma of addiction and mental illness in healthcare: the case of patients' experiences in dental settings. PLoS One 2017;12(5). https://doi.org/10.1371/journal.pone.0177388.

24. Armstrong D, Orr M, Judith. This dentist broke his opioid habit. Can the dental profession do the same? STAT. Available at: https://www.statnews.com/2017/02/ 14/dentists-opioid-prescribing/. Accessed January 8, 2020.

25. Available at: https://legiscan.com/MA/bill/H238/2019. Accessed January 8, 2020.

26. Mcpherson C, Boyne H, Willis R. The role of family in residential treatment patient retention. Int J Ment Health Addict 2016;15(4):933–41.

27. Ventura AS, Bagley SM. To improve substance use disorder prevention, treatment and recovery. J Addict Med 2017;11(5):339–41.

28. Difranza JR, Bhuvaneswar C, Jolicoeur D, et al. Tobacco use disorder. J Addict Med 2016;10(3):143–7.

29. Basu G, Phillips Costa V, Jain P. Clinicians obligations to use qualified medical interpreters when caring for patients with limited english proficiency. AMA J Ethics 2017;19(3):245–52.

30. Centers for Disease Control and Prevention.CDC guideline for prescribing opioids for chronic pain. Available at: https://www.cdc.gov/drugoverdose/prescribing/guideline.html. Accessed January 26, 2020.
31. Centers for Disease Control and Prevention. What states need to know about PDMPs. Available at: https://www.cdc.gov/drugoverdose/pdmp/states.html. Accessed January 26, 2020.
32. Zhang B, Bondy SJ, Diemert LM. Can dentists help patients quit smoking ?: the role of cessation medications. Dent News 2017;24(2):46–55.
33. Knapp E, Mitchell A, Riccelli A, et al. Effect on dental hygiene students of a substance use imulation conducted with nursing students. J Dent Educ 2018;82(5): 469–74.
34. Davis S, Shenson J, Chen Q, et al. Growth of secure messaging through a patient portal as a form of outpatient interaction across clinical specialties. Appl Clin Inform 2015;06(02):288–304.
35. Parish CL, Pereyra MR, Pollack HA, et al. Screening for substance misuse in the dental care setting: findings from a nationally representative survey of dentists. Addiction 2015;110(9):1516–23.
36. Patient-Reported Outcomes Measurement Information System (PROMIS). National Institute on Aging. Available at: https://www.nia.nih.gov/research/resource/patient-reported-outcomes-measurement-information-system-promis. Accessed January 26, 2020.
37. Patient Gateway. Massachusetts General Hospital. Available at: https://www.massgeneral.org/services/patient-gateway. Accessed January 26, 2020.
38. Estai M, Kruger E, Tennant M, et al. Challenges in the uptake of telemedicine in dentistry. Rural Remote Health 2016;16(4):3915.

# Special High-Risk Populations in Dentistry

## The Adolescent Patient, the Elderly Patient, and the Woman of Childbearing Age

Jennifer Magee, DMD, MPH[a],*, Britta E. Magnuson, DMD[b],
Donavon Khosrow K. Aroni, DMD, MS[c]

### KEYWORDS

- Vulnerable populations • Substance use • Adolescents
- Women of childbearing age • Older adults

### KEY POINTS

- The dental provider plays a key role in the care of special populations and must work in coordination with other medical professionals to provide optimal, individualized care.
- Nonjudgmental patient–provider relationships are important to establishing trust and facilitate asking difficult questions.
- Setting expectations for pain and discussing the alternatives, risks, and benefits of treatment options is an aspect of best practices.
- Dental professional need to consider the risk of misuse and abuse, including diversion, of medications in these special populations.

## INTRODUCTION

The dental provider plays an important role in the treatment of special populations of patients, including adolescents, women of childbearing age, and the elderly. Although these groups may seem very different, they share characteristics that require special consideration by the dental provider, especially when prescribing pain medications. Providers best serve these patients by recognizing the unique needs and offering individualized, compassionate, and comprehensive care, in collaboration with their medical colleagues.

Treatment of any patient must begin with a comprehensive evaluation. This evaluation provides an opportunity to build trust and to recognize any areas that may

[a] MGH Dental Group – Danvers, Department of Oral Surgery, Harvard School of Dental Medicine, 104 Endicott Street, Suite 101, Danvers, MA 01923, USA; [b] Department of Diagnostic Sciences, Tufts University School of Dental Medicine, 1 Kneeland Street, Boston, MA 02111, USA; [c] Division of Craniofacial Pain and Headache, Tufts University School of Dental Medicine, 1 Kneeland Street, Boston, MA 02111, USA
* Corresponding author.
E-mail address: jamagee@partners.org

Dent Clin N Am 64 (2020) 585–595
https://doi.org/10.1016/j.cden.2020.02.007
0011-8532/20/© 2020 Elsevier Inc. All rights reserved.

require further discussion, and those that may require consultation with other medical professionals. A thorough review of the medical history should include a discussion of medical issues, past surgeries and hospitalizations, current medications, and known drug allergies. Discussion of past dental experiences, concerns, and areas that are worrisome to the patient can help to identify triggers that may make the patient uncomfortable. This time is ideal time to discuss psychosocial issues, including substance abuse concerns, support at home, and other pressures that may prevent the patient from fully engaging in the recommended treatment.

A critical first step in developing this dentist–patient relationship is creating an open and safe environment that facilitates honest discussion. Providers who are comfortable with exploring all topics during the initial examination and gathering a history are more likely to elicit honest responses from the patient. Adopting a nonjudgmental approach may help to put the patient at ease, increasing the likelihood of full disclosure of information regarding health history, social pressures, and any history of substance abuse or misuse. Dental providers who see this process as an aspect of their professional role are more likely to ask patients about these sensitive topics.[1]

The development of a treatment plan should include focus on comprehensive care whenever possible, and the establishment of a "dental home" is important for the development adequate longitudinal care. Patients with special health care needs and vulnerable populations benefit from additional support to ensure that they have the resources to keep their appointments. Providing a supportive environment may provide sufficient incentive to encourage the patient to continue with needed treatment.

Including patients in treatment planning helps to support their feeling of autonomy and helps to clarify their priorities. A discussion of the risks, benefits, and alternatives in treatment should include the expectation of discomfort, the need for pain medication, and the desires of the patient. An explanation of procedures before performing them can help the patient to feel a greater sense of control and set the expectation for reasonable discomfort and a realistic timeline for healing. Honest and open discussion regarding the level of pain expected will lead to a discussion pertaining to prescriptions and contribute to boundary setting. There is an ethical obligation to treat pain, but the patient must be aware that the goal is not to treat until there is no pain; rather, treatment should continue to a point at which the patient believes his or her pain is at a reasonable level. This understanding may decrease the need for pain medication and the duration for which it is needed.

Patients should be encouraged to establish care with all necessary medical and mental health providers, and to adhere to recommended treatment and follow-up visits. Explaining the role of oral health in overall health, as well as the ways medical issues and medications impact oral health, may help the patient to recognize the role of the dentist in complete health maintenance. If patients mention not taking medication or following through with advice as recommended, it is helpful to follow-up and encourage them to speak to their physician without managing their medications on their own.

For the provider, it is important to have positive relationships with other local medical professionals to establish a referral network. Comfort in speaking to medical colleagues is an important tool in providing the best care possible for patients. Incorporating medical care and follow-up as part of the patient's overall plan demonstrates the importance of such to the patient and allows the dental provider to be aware of the concerns of their medical colleagues.

The need to evaluate the risks and benefits of the prescribed pain medications in these special populations is substantial and can help to inform the decision of which medications to prescribe, as well as the dosage and duration of the prescription. We now have a better understanding of the risks of prescription pain medications, which relates to the ethical obligation to provide appropriate pain relief. The tenet of prescribing the lowest level appropriate to reach the desired effect is an important one, especially in these higher risk groups.

## ASKING DIFFICULT QUESTIONS

Knowing how to address sensitive topics is a necessary skill for all health care providers. Avoiding uncomfortable topics is likely to prevent a provider from learning important information that is key to the appropriate treatment of the patient. Psychosocial issues, such as family dynamics, safety, and drug and alcohol experience should be tantamount to the exploration of commonly explored medical issues, such as a family history of heart disease or diabetes. Establishing an open and nonjudgmental environment can lead to a discussion in which a patient is willing to disclose information that is critical to proper diagnosis and development of an ideal treatment plan.

Another important part of asking difficult questions is being self-aware as a provider, recognizing one's own triggers and issues, and avoiding bringing one's own preconceived notions into the conversation. It is important to stay emotionally neutral to keep the discussion focused on the patient. Taking time to recognize and address one's own concerns outside of the encounter will allow the dental provider more freedom when speaking to his or her patients.

## ADHERENCE

Adequately explaining a treatment plan to the patient, and the way ancillary treatments play into it, is essential. After evaluating the patient and determining treatment options, careful consideration of whether his or her pain can be treated by alternative sources is necessary. This process should include a discussion with the patient regarding the expected course of recovery, symptoms about which the patient should be concerned, and pain relief options based on current best practices. The setting of expectations is beneficial to both the patient and the provider.

There may be some resistance from patients if they feel the recommended course of treatment will not be adequate. Accordingly, the use of guidelines, when available, is a helpful tool to reassure the patient and allow the clinician to maintain best practices. The use of a patient contract may be considered to formalize the expected behaviors, treatment, and follow-up. Any time there is concern relating to language, literacy, or cultural limitations, additional resources should be used.

Comprehensive dental care is a lifelong commitment that should be stressed to the patient. Follow-up with medical colleagues and, if needed, addiction referrals, should be encouraged.

## ASSESSING RISK FACTORS

Special populations are at risk of harm associated with potential misuse of medications, as well as diversion of their medications for nonmedical use by others. Diversion of medication is the redirection from the intended, lawful use for which it was prescribed to another person for a use unintended by the prescriber. This unlawful use may be due to family, societal, or economic pressures.[2] Patients may keep excess medication just in case, which is a potential problem because someone may find it and use it for nonmedical purposes. Patients have reported using pain medication to trade for other medications or asking for a prescription so they can give it to family members who either use it themselves or sell it.[2]

An important way to decrease diversion is through education of the patient by the provider.[3] Education to better understand the harms of excess prescription opioids, help to recognize the signs of misuse, and consider potential for diversion is essential. Appreciating the value of the medication for nonmedical use and therefore the incentive of some patients to misrepresent pain to obtain prescription medication in excess of what is needed is important to understanding the problem. The use of checklists by providers, such as the Controlled Substance Risk Mitigation checklist, can help dental professionals to better evaluate a patient's potential for abuse. Increasing physician awareness in these areas may encourage altering dosages before writing a prescription for an opioid.

Although there is no indication that emotional trauma is a proximate cause of substance abuse, the relationship between post-traumatic stress disorder (PTSD), substance use disorders,[4,5] and treatment-resistant pain conditions is well-established.[6] In another article in this special issue, the authors address the issue of PTSD and substance abuse risk in greater depth. Women are twice as likely to experience trauma-related PTSD than men, with co-occurring rates of substance use disorder ranging from 25% to 50%. In a recent study with a large population sample, subjects having clinical PTSD had a 2.56-fold increase in joint pain,[7] and a meta-analysis has confirmed the strong relationship between various chronic pain conditions and PTSD.[6] The role of central sensitization is most commonly discussed as an underlying mechanism with respect to the relationship between chronic pain and trauma, although there remains a debate regarding clear causation. Kindler and colleagues[7] argue that their results "should encourage general practitioners and dentists to acknowledge the role of PTSD and traumatic events in the diagnosis and therapy of TMD, especially in a period of international migration and military foreign assignments." Given high rates of co-occurrence with substance use disorders, we similarly reason that a thorough assessment should address substance use risk, while acknowledging PTSD as a significant comorbid risk factor.

## THE ADOLESCENT PATIENT

Adolescence is a transitional phase between childhood and adulthood that is marked by a growing sense of independence from parents or guardians. Adolescence is a time when individuals engage in more risk-taking behavior, which is thought to be due to the maturing brain's reward centers developing faster than the control centers. Caring for adolescent patients requires an understanding of the biologic and emotional changes that the adolescent undergoes, to provide appropriate guidance and support as a health care provider. The establishment of a trusting relationship, asking direct questions regarding drug and alcohol use, engagement with parents or guardians, and, when needed, referral to other medical resources are particularly important during this developmental phase.

As the adolescent works to establish autonomy, there are legal and ethical limitations regarding to what they can consent on their own. Conversations and decision making should involve the parents or guardians if the patient is under 18, or if the patient is 18 or older and wishes to have parents present. Adolescent 18 years and older must consent to discussion of their care, regardless of whether they are still on their parents' insurance or if parents are paying for their care. Even for minor patients, it is helpful to have a private conversation to allow for disclosure of a history of substance use regarding which they do not want their parents to know. Assumptions should not be made about an adolescent's support system, and offering support from sources outside the family may be helpful in cases of suspected family problems with substance abuse.

Support systems play a crucial role during all stages of life, but adolescents are particularly vulnerable to the impact of their home life. During the teen years, a growing sense of independence often means that adolescent patients are more likely to be responsible for their own medication management, making nonmedical use more likely.[8] Engaging parents or guardians in the process and clearly defining the expectation that the parent or guardian maintains responsibility for securing and dispensing medications may decrease the potential for nonmedical use or diversion. Families should be encouraged to have discussions regarding their own expectations relating to nonmedical opioid use, so the adolescent has clear boundaries regarding what constitutes safe and acceptable behavior.

Some adolescents may not have strong support systems at home and may benefit from referral to community resources for social work services, mental health providers, or addiction support organizations. Teens who have experienced a caregiver with substance abuse are considered at higher risk of substance abuse themselves, as well as mental health issues and accidental overdose.[9] Substance use during adolescence may limit the quality of social interactions, leading to isolation and deterioration of support systems.[10]

Dental providers should question changes in appearance, disorientation, erratic behavior, changes in pupil size, and injuries to the teeth or soft tissues as possible signs of substance abuse. Initial signs of mental illness may occur during adolescence, so sensitivity to such is important, because it may present in various forms. Findings of concern should be discussed with the patient in an open and honest fashion, and include discussion with parents or guardians as well as consideration of referral to other medical professionals, if needed.

It is important to recognize that prescription opioid medication for a dental procedure such as a third molar extraction may represent the initial exposure for an adolescent, and use before high school graduation has been associated with a 33% greater risk of subsequent misuse.[11] Interestingly, this correlation is particularly strong in adolescents without histories of drug use, and among those who have negative feelings regarding illegal drug use.[11] This finding highlights the importance of comprehensive counseling of patients and families regarding the dangers of nonmedical prescription drug use, which may not be initially clear to them. Although a majority of patients who reported nonmedical use of prescription opioids while in high school no longer reported it within 3 years,[8] the high abuse potential of these medications and risk of diversion makes judicious prescribing to this group imperative.

There are no absolute indicators of which adolescents are at highest risk of prescription opioid abuse, although it has been linked to heavy alcohol and marijuana use.[8] Therefore, screening questions that are sensitive to adolescents should assess past use of alcohol and drugs, as well as potential opioid abuse risk. Allowing screening questions to be answered anonymously and without the involvement of parents has been shown to increase responsiveness.[12] The use of alcohol and marijuana increases the likelihood of nonmedical use of prescription opioids,[8] so positive responses regarding such should prompt increased counseling if an opioid prescription is deemed necessary.

If an adolescent presents with pain or will be undergoing a procedure that will likely cause discomfort, opioid alternatives should be considered first. Although risk assessment of abuse potential is critical in determining which medications to prescribe, it is important to first familiarize oneself with what is appropriate in the clinical situation.

Nonopioid management should be attempted whenever reasonable. If opioids are deemed most appropriate to treat pain, then the provider must have a frank conversation with the patient to discuss the purpose of the medication, the goals of use, and abuse potential, and warn against using the medication for nonmedical reasons or sharing the medication. Additionally, more frequent follow-up is recommended as an element of the treatment plan.

## WOMEN OF CHILDBEARING AGE

Women of childbearing age, approximately from 18 years to 44 years of age, offer unique challenges relating to prescribing pain medications. This age range corresponds with a time in a woman's life when she is most likely to develop an addiction. It is also a period during which she is most likely to become pregnant, planned, unplanned, or unknown, which must be considered when prescribing medications that could be detrimental to a developing fetus. Careful medical history taking and asking about changes in health and possible pregnancy are important. Women should be encouraged to seek routine medical care especially if they are, or suspect they might be, pregnant.

Pregnancy can be a challenging time for a woman and those with a history of trauma may struggle with a range of increased medical concerns, exacerbation of pain conditions, as well as worsening of some psychiatric disorders.[4] Creating a warm, welcoming, and nonjudgmental environment for treatment will make patients more comfortable and increase the likelihood that they will return for care. Medical care and follow-up during pregnancy are very important to ensuring a healthy baby and expectant mother; asking about recent medical visits and encouraging compliance with the obstetrician's recommendations should be part of every dental visit.

Woman of childbearing age with substance abuse disorders are much more likely to have an unplanned pregnancy and receive less prenatal care,[13] making this an important consideration in prescribing pain medication to this group of patients. Careful questioning and education to ensure they understand the risks of not disclosing a possible pregnancy is important when determining the class of medication to prescribe in this group.[14–16] The question of pregnancy status is often and easily asked when taking dental radiographs; a similar approach can be used for this purpose.

Substance use during pregnancy is not rare, with national reporting indicating more than 8% of US pregnant women "using an illicit substance in the past 30 days."[9] Pharmacy data indicate that approximately 20% of pregnant women on Medicaid and almost 15% of pregnant women with private insurance filled a prescription for opioids in the previous year,[17] suggesting that opioids are frequently used as a means to manage pain in this patient population.

Extended opioid use in pregnancy can lead to an increased risk of congenital malformation.[17] Continued use of opioids in pregnancy increases the risk of neonatal abstinence syndrome, a complex condition resulting from the cessation of drug exposure after birth. The syndrome can present as irritability and excessive crying, feeding issues, hyperthermia, and, less commonly, seizures.[18–20] The mechanism is not well-understood, although it is thought to be due to changes in dopamine, norepinephrine, and serotonin in these babies who have prenatal exposure to opioids.[19] There are many prenatal maternal behaviors that are thought to impact the presentation of the newborn, including the specific substance and duration of use, treatment, or opioid substitution program participation, and degree of compliance with prenatal care.[19] There is no standard treatment for these babies, although treatment generally includes the provision of a calm environment and frequent feedings to decrease hunger.[19]

Women using opioids while pregnant may be able to participate in an opioid substitution program, which will not eliminate the risk of neonatal abstinence syndrome, yet can decrease the riskier behaviors associated with drug seeking and allow for increased compliance with routine medical care.[19] Opioid agonist therapy, such as methadone or buprenorphine, is considered preferable compared with complete cessation because it decreases withdrawal symptoms and chances of relapse; however, it must be managed by addiction specialists trained in pregnancy, which may be difficult to find in medically underserved areas.

Although adherence to prenatal care and participation in substance abuse treatment may seem like obvious choices for an expectant mother, the legal ramifications can be overwhelming for some women.[18] Many states consider drug use during pregnancy, including opioid substitution programs, to constitute child abuse. In these states, a woman using opioids is more likely to have a child removed from her care.[9] Treatment options for dependence during pregnancy are crucially important, yet there is a lack of treatment facilities available for these patients. Sadly, those with fewer resources and reduced socioeconomic status tend to have the most difficult time finding highly specialized care, despite their high-risk status.[17]

Dental providers should question changes in appearance, disorientation, erratic behavior, injuries to the teeth or soft tissues, and drug-seeking behavior as possible signs of substance abuse. Concerning findings should be discussed with the patient in an open and honest fashion, as well as consideration of referral to other medical professionals, if necessary.

Pregnancy can be a challenging time in a woman's life, and those with substance abuse issues, or risk factors, warrant additional attention. Sharing the dental diagnosis and recommended treatment with the patient and allowing her to participate in treatment planning demonstrates respect for her autonomy and encourages compliance. An open discussion regarding the expected discomfort and pain relief options that can be offered may help to decrease the need for prescription pain medication. When medication does need to be prescribed, it should be done carefully and in conjunction with obstetrician clearance. Before performing any dental work, a consultation with the physician is recommended; this step will also illuminate whether the pregnant patient is actually under the care of a physician. If a pregnant patient has not sought prenatal care or has not been seen recently, the dental professional provides a vital service by insisting on examination with an obstetrician before proceeding.

## OLDER ADULTS

Medical advances and lifestyle changes have resulted in a longer life expectancy, with almost 15% of Americans currently over the age of 65.[21,22] There are physiologic and emotional changes as we age that need to be taken into consideration for treatment of this population. Sixty percent of older adults manage 2 or more chronic conditions.[23,24] In addition to other medical considerations, a provider must also consider the medications used to treat them and how that impacts dental care. In response to a growing concern regarding the long-term impact of nonsteroidal anti-inflammatory drug use and potential for undertreatment of pain in the elderly, there was a shift toward opioid prescriptions, leading to a doubling of opioid prescriptions in older adults between 1999 and 2010, with 10% of clinic visits for older adults involving prescription of an opioid.[25]

Dental treatment of the elderly can be very complex. The aging process, which is associated with taking more medications, often results in a decrease in the quantity and quality of saliva. This factor, combined with heavily restored dentition and potential issues with dexterity and brushing, can lead to a decline in the state of oral health and the need for significant dental procedures. Even patients who previously had few dental needs can find themselves with a failing dentition if care is not taken to avoid the problem. The financial ramifications can present an additional challenge to those on fixed incomes.

Older adults should be connected with a primary care doctor to help manage the complexities of aging, and may consider someone specializing in geriatric medicine, if available in their area. Confirmation that all medications are being taken as prescribed should be a routine part of every dental visit, as well as asking about changes in health, recent hospitalizations, and any falls. Inquiring regarding these issues reaffirms to patients that they are important concerns and need to be discussed and followed up with any health care provider. It can be helpful to encourage older patients to maintain a written or typed list of current medications and names of their physicians.

Mobility and ambulation are concerns for the elderly, especially given the morbidity and mortality associated with injuries from falls, which are more common, independent of opioid use.[26] Prescription medications that may alter the patient's balance or decision making should be approached with caution. Inappropriate or excessive use of opioids have been found to result in an increased risk of injury,[27] especially for the elderly with new opioid prescriptions.[26] The sedative side effect of medications should be discussed, especially for patients who continue to drive.[28] Careful, complete, and open discussions with these patients are important to assess and counsel regarding these risks, and for them to understand which areas are of greatest concern.

Elderly patients may require assistance from family or friends, and an open discussion of their support network should occur at the first visit and be reviewed when there is a change in health or life events, such as moving or the death of a spouse. Patients should be encouraged to discuss challenges at home, especially pertaining to dexterity required for oral health home care or taking medications, as well as concerns regarding safety in the home. Elder abuse is a serious issue, which may be viewed as physical or emotional abuse or as neglect. It may include withholding or diversion of medications, both for medical conditions and pain relief. Many states have reporting requirements if elder abuse is suspected. Providing local resources for the elderly can help them to take advantage of local community offerings for older adults that may help them to access the services and connection that they need.

Physiologic changes with aging may include changes in drug absorption, metabolism, and excretion. These changes may be augmented or enhanced by disease processes or other medications. Thorough accessing of health history and discussion may illuminate areas that the patient has forgotten to disclose. For example, it is important that the dental provider has a complete list of current medications that are each linked back to a medical condition being treated. Medical consultation with the patient's physician is encouraged when there is any question of the patient's ability to be an accurate health historian. A discussion of health history and the treatment plan with a family member may be helpful, but can only occur with the express permission of the patient, unless there is a legal finding that an older individual is no longer competent to make his or her own medical decisions.

Patients may experience an increase in pain as they age owing to many factors, including neuropathic, musculoskeletal, inflammatory, and mechanical/compressive.[28] Given the complex causes of pain in the elderly, there should be open discussions regarding the objective that treating the pain may not lead to complete relief, but rather a decrease to a level less likely to impact independence and quality of life. In general, pain in the elderly is best treated with acetaminophen and nonmedication options, such as physical therapy, whenever possible.[29] When there is no option other than opioids, it is best to stick to those with the shortest duration of action and at the lowest effective dose.[30]

Sudden mental status changes can occur owing to a variety of causes and are not considered a normal part of aging. Dementia is not well-understood, but there is some evidence that opioids may increase the risk of developing it over time.[31] Cognitive decline and confusion are potential issues and must be considered in choosing medications to prescribe and the possible impact they may have directly on the patient or through drug–drug interactions. Changes in the way the body metabolizes medication as we age may result in overmedication, often resulting in confusion. If a significant change has been noted in an established patient, a consultation with his or her physician is warranted immediately.

There is a decreased risk of death owing to opioid overdose in the elderly[30] that, along with the perceived decreased risk of addiction and the multiple medical issues that may result in pain, results in elderly people being more likely to fill an opioid prescription.[27] However, nonmedical opioid use was found to be associated with a greater rate of alcohol abuse and mental health conditions.[27] The elderly population is more likely than the general population to receive prescriptions for longer duration and at higher doses.[27] Patients in long-term care facilities are especially vulnerable to the misperception that opioids are not harmful to the elderly.[32]

Dental providers should question changes in appearance, disorientation, erratic behavior, injuries to the teeth or soft tissue, and increased reports of falls or injuries as possible signs of substance abuse. Concerning findings should be discussed with the older patient in an open and honest manner, as well as consideration of referral to other medical professionals, if appropriate.

Elderly patients benefit from comprehensive dental care, and when they present with pain, a proper diagnosis is a necessary first step. Once a treatment plan is developed, the expectation of discomfort can be determined and a prescription can be provided, if necessary. Despite concerns with opioid prescriptions in this population, when used appropriately they serve an important role in improving quality of life. Short-term, appropriate use can decrease pain and improve sleep in the elderly.[33,34]

## SUMMARY

Comprehensive and compassionate treatment of vulnerable patients is an important service to the community, although dental treatment of special populations can represent a challenge. The dental provider must be able to recognize the issues surrounding substance use/abuse, coordinate care with medical providers and build a trusting provider-patient relationship to achieve success. Open conversations regarding expectations of pain, and the risks, benefits and alternatives to opioids are important aspects of the best care of these patients.

## DISCLOSURE

Partial support was received for the preparation of this article through a grant from "The Coverys Community Healthcare Foundation".

## REFERENCES

1. Parish CL, Pereyra MR, Pollack HA, et al. Screening for substance misuse in the dental care setting: findings from a nationally representative survey of dentists. Addiction 2015;110(9):1516–23.

2. Green T, Bowman S, Ray M, et al. Collaboration or Coercion? Partnering to divert prescription opioid medications. J Urban Health 2013;90(4):758–67.

3. Inciardi J, Surratt H, Cicero T, et al. Prescription opioid abuse and diversion in an urban community: the results of an ultrarapid assessment. Pain Med 2009;10(3): 537–48.

4. Banerjee S, Spry C. Concurrent treatment for substance use disorder and trauma-related comorbidities: a review of clinical effectiveness and guidelines. Canadian Agency for Drugs and Technologies in Health; 2017.

5. Gradus J. Prevalence and prognosis of stress disorders: a review of the epidemiologic literature. Clin Epidemiol 2017;9:251–60.

6. Siqveland J, Hussain A, Lindstrøm JC, et al. Prevalence of posttraumatic stress disorder in persons with chronic pain: a meta-analysis. Front Psychiatry 2017; 8:164.

7. Kindler S, Schwahn C, Bernhardt O, et al. Association between symptoms of posttraumatic stress disorder and signs of temporomandibular disorders in the general population. J Oral Facial Pain Headache 2019;33(1):67–76.

8. Mccabe SE, Schulenberg JE, Omalley PM, et al. Non-medical use of prescription opioids during the transition to adulthood: a multi-cohort national longitudinal study. Addiction 2013;109(1):102–10.

9. Winstanley EL, Stover AN. The impact of the opioid epidemic on children and adolescents. Clin Ther 2019;41(9):1655–62.

10. Moore SK, Grabinski M, Bessen S, et al. Web-based prescription opioid abuse prevention for adolescents: program development and formative evaluation. JMIR Form Res 2019;3(3):e1169–77.

11. Miech R, Johnston L, Omalley PM, et al. Prescription opioids in adolescence and future opioid misuse. Pediatrics 2015;136(5):e1169–77.

12. Chavez LJ, Bradley KA, Lapham GT, et al. Identifying problematic substance use in a national sample of adolescents using frequency questions. J Am Board Fam Med 2019;32(4):550–8.

13. Kocherlakota. Neonatal abstinence syndrome. Pediatrics 2014;134(2):e547–61.

14. Maeda A, Bateman B, Clancy C, et al. Opioid abuse and dependence during pregnancy. Obstet Anesth Dig 2015;35(4):191–2.

15. Martin EB, Mazzola NM, Brandano J, et al. Clinicians' recognition and management of emotions during difficult healthcare conversations. Patient Educ Couns 2015;98(10):1248–54.

16. Rhee T. Coprescribing of benzodiazepines and opioids in older adults: rates, correlates, and national trends. J Gerontol A Biol Sci Med Sci 2019;74(12):1910–5.

17. Desai RJ, Hernandez-Diaz S, Bateman BT, et al. Increase in prescription opioid use during pregnancy among Medicaid-enrolled women. Obstet Gynecol 2014; 123(5):997–1002.

18. Krans E, Patrick S. Opioid use disorder in pregnancy: health policy and practice in the midst of an epidemic. Obstet Gynecol 2016;128(1):4–10.

19. Stover MW, Davis JM. Opioids in pregnancy and neonatal abstinence syndrome. Semin Perinatol 2015;39(7):561–5.

20. Kozhimannil KB, Graves AJ, Levy R, et al. Nonmedical us of prescription opioids among pregnant US women. Womens Health Issues 2017;27(3):308–15.

21. Fain K, Alexander G, Dore D, et al. Frequency and predictors of analgesic prescribing in U.S. nursing home residents with persistent pain. J Am Geriatr Soc 2016;65(2):286–93.

22. Gerlach L, Olfson M, Kales H, et al. Opioids and other central nervous system-active polypharmacy in older adults in the United States. J Am Geriatr Soc 2017;65(9):2052–6.

23. Available at: https://www.healthypeople.gov/2020/topics-objectives/topic/older-adults/. Accessed August 6, 2019.

24. Saia, Schiff, Wachman, et al. Caring for pregnant women with opioid use disorder in the USA: explaining and improving treatment. Curr Obstet Gynecol Rep 2016; 5(3):257–63.

25. Steinman M, Komaiko K, Fung K, et al. Use of opioids and other analgesics by older adults in the United States, 1999–2010. Pain Med 2015;16(2):319–27.

26. Krebs E, Paudel M, Taylor B, et al. Association of opioids with falls, fractures, and physical performance among older men with persistent musculoskeletal pain. J Gen Intern Med 2016;31(5):463–9.

27. Carter M, Yang B, Davenport M, et al. Increasing rates of opioid misuse among older adults visiting emergency departments. Innov Aging 2019;3(1):igz002.

28. Galicia-Castillo M. Opioids for persistent pain in older adults. Cleve Clin J Med 2016;83(6):443–51.

29. Makris U, Abrams R, Gurland B, et al. Management of persistent pain in the older patient. JAMA 2014;312(8):825.

30. Naples J, Gellad W, Hanlon J. The role of opioid analgesics in geriatric pain management. Clin Geriatr Med 2016;32(4):725–35.

31. Swart L, van der Zanden V, Spies P, et al. The comparative risk of delirium with different opioids: a systematic review. Drugs Aging 2017;34(6):437–43.

32. Griffioen C, Willems E, Kouwenhoven S, et al. Physicians' knowledge of and attitudes toward use of opioids in long-term care facilities. Pain Pract 2016;17(5): 625–32.

33. Papaleontiou M, Henderson C Jr, Turner B, et al. Outcomes associated with opioid use in the treatment of chronic noncancer pain in older adults: a systematic review and meta-analysis. J Am Geriatr Soc 2010;58(7):1353–69.

34. Available at: http://www.aapd.org/research/oral-health-policies–recommendations/ substance-abuse-in-adolescent-patients/. Accessed July 1, 2019.

# Opioid Prescribing in Dental Practice: Managing Liability Risks

David A. Keith, BDS, FDSRCS, DMD[a,*], Ronald J. Kulich, PhD[b,c,d], Alexis A. Vasciannie[e], Richard S. Harold, DMD, JD[f]

## KEYWORDS

- Safe prescribing • Controlled substances • Pain management • Opioids
- Dental Practice

## KEY POINTS

- Dentistry has been on the forefront of acute pain management for more than 200 years, and continues to have an obligation to focus on "rational prescribing" with their patients.
- The opioid use crisis and concerns over controlled substance risk have changed practice patterns throughout health care.
- As the role of dentistry has expanded, dentists have an increasing obligation to assess and mitigate risk for their patients, and regulatory agencies are increasingly mandating strategies for risk assessment.
- Common violations of legal and regulatory requirements made by practicing dentists are reviewed, and strategies to maximize safe prescribing practices are outlined.

## INTRODUCTION

From a public policy perspective, past dental practice patterns have had an impact on the opioid epidemic. In one of the earlier conferences on controlled substance risk within the practice of dentistry, Denisco and colleagues[1] concluded that "dentists cannot assume that their prescribing of opioids does not affect the opioid abuse problem in the United States." The American Dental Association's (ADA's) recent policy on opioid prescribing[2] focuses on the important role in dentistry with respect to minimizing the impact of the opioid crisis. In response to these recommendations,

[a] Oral and Maxillofacial Surgery, Massachusetts General Hospital, Harvard School of Dental Medicine, Fruit Street, Warren 1201, Boston, MA 02114, USA; [b] Tufts University School of Dental Medicine, Craniofacial Pain & Headache Center, 1 Kneeland Street, Boston, MA 02111, USA; [c] Department of Anesthesia, Critical Care and Pain Medicine, Massachusetts General Hospital, Boston, MA, USA; [d] Department of Psychiatry, Massachusetts General Hospital, Boston, MA, USA; [e] Department of Diagnostic Sciences, Tufts University School of Dental Medicine, 1 Kneeland Street, Boston, MA 02111, USA; [f] Department of Comprehensive Care, Tufts University School of Dental Medicine, 1 Kneeland Street, Boston, MA 02111, USA
* Corresponding author.
*E-mail address:* DKEITH@mgh.harvard.edu

Dent Clin N Am 64 (2020) 597–608
https://doi.org/10.1016/j.cden.2020.03.003
0011-8532/20/© 2020 Elsevier Inc. All rights reserved.

dentists need to understand the legal, regulatory, and ethical environment surrounding dental pain management. As the nature and characteristics of the prescription opioid crisis have evolved, so do the legal and regulatory parameters. Hence, dentists need to keep abreast of advances in pain management practices and policies and guidelines.

## HISTORY OF OPIOIDS AND PAIN MANAGEMENT

Prescribing patterns for the management of acute pain have changed over the years, ranging from extreme conservatism following the passage of the Harrison Narcotic Act in 1914,[3] which for the first time in US history made the possession of opioid-containing medications illegal without a prescription, to the period of liberal opioid prescribing beginning in the 1990s. At that time, pain specialists and advocacy groups began to complain that government regulations, policies, and pain management guidelines presented barriers to adequate pain relief. As a result, a dramatic increase in demand for prescription opioids occurred, and by 2010, opioid prescribing had increased dramatically with corresponding increases in overdoses and deaths. As a consequence of the current opioid crisis, government and regulatory agencies are now paying close attention to prescribing practices, and this increased scrutiny is affecting the dental profession as well.[4]

All prescribers have a responsibility to minimize the potential for drug misuse and diversion while maintaining legitimate access to opioids for patients in need of such analgesic treatment.,[1,5,6] The ADA statement[6] on the use of opioids in the treatment of dental pain recommends that dentists reduce the need for "just-in-case" prescriptions for dental pain. The statement covers the complexities of modern pain management in dentistry, including the nature of drug addiction, ways to screen patients for potential substance use disorders, and techniques for motivating at-risk individuals to seek appropriate treatment. Additional recommendations of the ADA include following the US Centers for Disease Control and Prevention (CDC) opioid prescribing guidelines[7] for chronic pain when appropriate, using their state's Prescription Drug Monitoring Program database, completing continuing education, and prescribing nonopioids as the first-line therapy for acute dental pain. The ADA supports statutory limits on opioid dosage and duration of no more than 7 days for the treatment of acute pain, consistent with CDC evidence-based guidelines. The Association's position is that as a profession, dentists can still do more to keep opioids from becoming a potential source of harm. The ADA also promotes interprofessional cooperation by working together with physicians, pharmacists, and other health care professionals, policy makers, and the public.[6] Recent studies suggest that the specific issues currently facing the dental profession are the disproportionate number of opioid prescriptions written by dentists for teenagers and young adults who are at increased risk of developing substance abuse issues.[8] Dentists are the leading source of opioid prescribing for adolescents and young adults because they are most likely to present with third molar issues.[9] Often patients do not consume the entire prescription and a number of pills are left over and subject to diversion. The adherence with evidence-based guidelines recommending nonsteroidal anti-inflammatory drugs and acetaminophen as first-line analgesics, which are more effective than opioids, will help minimize diversion and opioid misuse.[10]

When required, the prescribing of opioids is appropriate only after risk assessment and cooperation with other medical disciplines. The basic principles of prescribing for the management of dental pain are outlined in **Box 1**.

| Box 1 |
| --- |
| **Guidelines for prescribing controlled substances for acute dental pain** |
| 1. Conduct a medical and dental history to determine current medications, potential drug interactions and history of substance abuse. |
| 2. Follow and continually review Centers for Disease Control and Prevention and state licensing board recommendations for safe opioid prescribing. |
| 3. Register with and use prescription drug monitoring programs (PDMPs) to promote the appropriate use of controlled substances for legitimate medical purposes, while deterring the misuse, abuse, and diversion of these substances. |
| 4. Have a discussion with the patient about responsibilities for preventing misuse, abuse, storage, and disposal of prescription opioids. |
| 5. Consider treatment options that use best practices to prevent exacerbation of or relapse of opioid misuse. |
| 6. Consider nonsteroidal anti-inflammatory analgesics or acetaminophen as the first-line therapy for acute pain management. |
| 7. Recognize multimodal pain strategies for management for acute postoperative pain as a means for sparing the need for opioid analgesics. |
| 8. Consider coordination with other treating clinicians, including pain specialists, when prescribing opioids for the management of chronic orofacial pain. |
| 9. Be aware that practicing in good faith and using professional judgment regarding the prescribing of opioids for the treatment of pain should not result in discipline for the willful and deceptive behavior of patients who successfully obtain opioids for nondental purposes. Good dental treatment records should support your prescribing decisions. |
| 10. Dental students, residents and practicing dentists, and dental hygienists are encouraged to seek continuing education in addictive disease and pain management as related to opioid prescribing. |
| *Adapted from* American Dental Association. Statement on the use of opioids in the treatment of dental pain. Available at: https://www.ada.org/en/advocacy/current-policies/substance-use-disorders. Copyright © 2005 American Dental Association. All rights reserved. Reprinted with permission. |

Despite adhering to these principles, the dentist may be subjected to manipulation, deception, or various types of prescription misuse by the patient, which could result in diversion of opioid pills. These actions come in different forms.

### Prescription Tampering

The use of written prescriptions represents a liability for the prescriber, as the script can be altered or forged. A survey from West Virginia documented the various ways that opioids can be illegally obtained in the dental practice[11] (see **Box 2**).

Electronic prescribing, allowing prescribers to electronically write prescriptions for controlled substances and permitting pharmacies to receive, dispense, and archive these e-prescriptions will help to curb these abuses. Electronic prescribing for controlled substances (EPCS) will also provide more robust audit trails and "identity proofing" responsibilities for prescribers and vendors. E-prescribing is legalized in all states and the District of Columbia with 82% of retail pharmacies fully enabled to accept these electronic prescriptions. E-prescribing is not mandated by the federal government; however, states are empowered to regulate prescribing. For example, in New York State, EPCS is required for both legal and controlled substances;

---

**Box 2**
**Strategies for illegally obtaining controlled substances**

- Fake pain symptoms: 43%
- Patient claims lost/stolen prescription: 28%
- Forged written prescription: 14%
- Altered pill number: 14%
- Fake prescription call-ins: 9%
- Stolen prescription pads: 9%
- Altered numbers on prescriptions: 9%

*Data from* Tufts Health Care Institute. Executive Summary: the role of dentists in preventing opioid abuse—Tufts Health Care Institute Program on Opioid Risk Management 12th Summit Meeting, March 11–12, 2010.

---

however, adoption has been slow because of implementation complexities. In Massachusetts, mandatory electronic prescribing has been delayed until January 1, 2021.[11–13]

The ADA has stated that dentists who are practicing in good faith and who use professional judgment in prescribing opioids for the treatment of dental pain should not be held responsible for the willful and deceptive behavior of patients. Dentists still need to be aware of these deceptive practices and make every effort to avoid the 2 most common deceptions: diversion and doctor shopping. Good treatment records documenting findings, diagnoses, and treatment plans will help support the dentist's decision to prescribe opioids when appropriate.

### Drug Diversion

*Drug diversion* is defined as the intentional transfer of a substance outside the guidelines set forth by the Food and Drug Administration (FDA), Drug Enforcement Administration (DEA), state licensing boards, and prescribing health care professionals.[14] Drug diversion is typically motivated by money or a substance use disorder. Controlled substances can be diverted at several steps along the course from manufacturer to patients and beyond.[15] (p2) Excessive prescribing contributes to drug diversion, as unused medications increase available inventory subject to potential abuse. Dentists are obligated to prescribe in a responsible manner, guarding against diversion while ensuring that patients have an adequate supply of analgesics for control of dental pain. Dental practices are targets for patients with substance use disorders who attempt to inappropriately obtain controlled substances for nondental purposes, creating a challenge to determine which patients are presenting for legitimate dental purposes and which are presenting with the conscious goal of feigning discomfort to obtain controlled substances.

### Doctor Shopping

*Doctor shopping* is a common technique used by patients whereby they frequent multiple providers complaining of the same problems to obtain multiple controlled substance prescriptions either for themselves or others. Although it is not possible for the dental practitioner to screen out all drug seekers, a thorough clinical examination, review of states' prescription drug monitoring programs (PDMPs) and documentation will help protect and support the dentist should scrutiny by the DEA, licensing authorities, or law enforcement occur. Strategies to mitigate risk should include documenting clinical and radiographic findings, asking patients for photo identification, and formulating a diagnosis and treatment plan, even if the treatment plan is as simple as referring to a specialist. Dental hygienists and other staff members are often an excellent source of information on patient drug-seeking behavior. An observant front desk receptionist may be in the best position to notice unusual or aberrant behavior and can pass this information along to the dentist.[15] [(p145-146)]

### Prescription Drug Monitoring Programs

PDMPs provide one of the most important vehicles for risk mitigation, and details of these programs are discussed in "Special Screening Resources: Strategies to Identify Substance Use Disorders, Including Opioid Misuse and Abuse" by Keith and Hernández-Nuño de la Rosa in this issue. The issue of liability for using or not using the PDMP databases has not been clearly defined in all jurisdictions and depends on the current laws of each state. Nonetheless, the prescribing dentist does have a duty to warn the patient about the adverse effects of the medications prescribed, and practice with reasonable care and in good faith when prescribing medications for pain control.[15,16]

PDMP databases can ensure safe and effective pain management for their patients. They also provide an excellent opportunity to discuss these risks with the patient. The dentist should check with their state dental societies and licensing boards for up-to-date information on applicable state regulations. Although prescribers are not required to obtain the patient's permission to access the PDMP in most states, it is recommended that the prescriber initiate a conversation with the patient, as well as cotreating, and the patient's other health care providers. If significant misuse or abuse is suspected about the PDMP search, dentists also are within their rights to contact the DEA or the local police department. As with all communications, patient care is maximized, and the dentist's risk is reduced when any of these actions are fully documented.

### DOCUMENTATION

Proper documentation is the professional and legal responsibility of all dental practitioners. Not only do dental records provide for continuity of care when treatment is transferred from one provider to another, but they provide a legal record to document that care has been provided according to professional standards. It is important to remember that judges, juries, dental board members, and lawyers maintain that "if it wasn't documented, it wasn't done." This policy applies to all visits, telephone conversations with patients and other care givers, prescriptions, and other clinically related issues. Accurate dental records are essential not only when documenting treatment but also when prescribing medications.[15] [(p171)] Typically, it is beneficial to record exact quotes from the patient, conversations with treating providers, and contacts with law enforcement.

Specific documentation for a controlled substance treatment plan also is essential. Some states require a *written informed consent* before prescribing opioids even for short-term treatment of acute dental pain. States are legislating the prescribing of opioids more frequently and more aggressively with limitations on the amount of medication that can be prescribed, and the steps prescribers need to take to avoid diversion. For example, Massachusetts requires that the PDMP be queried every time a Schedule II or III medication is prescribed and limits the quantity of an initial opioid prescriptions to a 7-day supply.[17] In addition, Massachusetts requires that dentists discuss substance abuse risks, disposal of unused medication, and the option to have prescriptions filled for fewer quantities when prescribing Schedule II medications. It is important to document in the patient treatment record that this discussion has taken place.

Treatment agreements addressing the clinician and patient rules for prescribing, using, and refilling controlled substances are common when opioids are written on a chronic basis. Although less common in dentistry, patients taking opioids under supervision of their primary care physician, pain specialist, or addiction specialist will have a controlled substance agreement in place. The general terms include provisions that the patient agrees to get prescriptions from only 1 prescriber; use 1 pharmacy; not use alcohol, other opioids, or illicit drugs or substances; submit to pill counts and random urine tests; and agree to participate in other treatments as indicated. If a patient has an agreement of this sort and requires dental surgery for which an opioid may be necessary, it is incumbent on the dentist to check with the primary prescriber to discuss a time-limited and dose-limited increase in opioids for the postoperative period.[18]

Dentists always practice "universal precautions" with respect to infection control. It is now strongly recommended that they adopt similar practice precautions when considering prescribing an opioid pain medication for a patient. The use of the Risk Assessment Checklist, as outlined in "Dentistry's Role in Assessing and Managing Controlled Substance Risk: Historical Overview, Current Barriers, and Working Toward Best Practices by Dhadwal and colleagues in this issue, ensures that all aspects of the decision-making process from initial examination and assessment to writing the prescription and subsequent follow-up are conducted in a safe, efficient, and responsible manner.

## DISPOSAL OF CONTROLLED SUBSTANCES

When prescribing controlled substances, many states now require practitioners to advise patients how to store and dispose of unused medications in a safe fashion. Most police stations and many pharmacies have disposal bins in their lobbies where the public may dispose of unused medication with no questions asked. The FDA has specific recommendations regarding the disposing of controlled substances.[19] The prescription bottle label should be removed or scratched out with a marker to cover up any identifying information.[15 (p153)]

## COMMON REGULATORY VIOLATIONS BY DENTAL PRACTITIONERS

Abuse, misuse, and diversion sometimes occur when dentists prescribe controlled substances for themselves, staff, family, or friends who are outside the scope of dentistry. Dental boards are known to discipline dentists for prescribing outside the scope of their practice even for antibiotics and cough and cold medication. Excessive prescribing of controlled substances even for patients of record, if not substantiated in patients' records, could result in serious consequences, including referral to the DEA.[15 (p170)] For those dentists personally suffering from a substance use disorder, the temptation to abuse one's prescribing privileges can have disastrous consequences.[20]

The DEA's mission is to enforce the controlled substances laws and regulations. The agency can initiate a practice inspection if a violation of these laws is suspected. Furthermore, a review of the dental practice's opioid prescribing history can become a part of a dental licensing board's inspection initiated as a result of other dental practice license violations (eg, infection control). Many states also require the dentist to complete biennial training on safe and effective opioid prescribing/pain management. Even if a dentist does not write prescriptions, Massachusetts requires that the dentist maintain a valid controlled substance state registration for the sole purpose of ordering/replenishing the emergency drug kit required for each dental office. It is each dentist's responsibility to know what is expected to comply with state and federal regulations.[19]

The best way to prepare for DEA or state licensing board inspections is to maintain accurate and comprehensive practice and dental treatment records that demonstrate that one has prescribed within the accepted standard of care. Should a dentist keep controlled substances in his or her office, regulatory agencies will want to be convinced that this is being done in a safe and secure manner. The DEA has a standing policy not to interfere with the doctor-patient relationship and dictate how providers prescribe. On the other hand, should a dentist be an outlier, that is, prescribing many more opioids than similar providers, or prescribing or giving refills without an examination, he or she will receive heightened scrutiny by the DEA. Dentists' treatment records should support their clinical decisions to prescribe. Care should be taken to document the findings, diagnosis, and treatment plans, and to assess pain levels and obtain informed consent when prescribing opioids. Although use and documentation of PDMP results is required in most states, the issue of liability for using or not using the PDMP databases has not been clearly defined in all jurisdictions. A brief review of the DEA Web site of cases that this agency brought against prescribers during 2004 to 2019 identifies a series of cases involving dentists. **Box 3** lists common issues reported in legal cases before the DEA. Details involving each individual case may vary. Some allegations involve illegal distribution and trafficking of controlled substances, record-keeping violations. money laundering, prescribing opioids for sex, and involvement in a "pill mill."[21] **Box 4** lists specific details for several complex cases that involved controlled substances and the practice of dentistry.

---

**Box 3**
**Common issues reported in legal cases**

- Prescribing dosages and amounts of controlled substances that were not justified based on the diagnoses and conditions documented.

- The dental records reflect deficiencies including lack of consistent intake history, few documented tests, lack of basis for diagnosis or rationale of treatment provided, lack of care coordination with primary care physicians and other specialists, lack of interval records documenting clinical progress, lack of documentation of discussion, or use of alternative therapies and regular comprehensive examinations, and lack of exit strategies from treatment with controlled substances.

- The dentist failed to take appropriate action when the patient breached his or her opioid contracts and ignored signs of addiction to controlled substances, billing insurance companies for complicated follow-up visits without justification in the clinical record.

- Treating patients and prescribing medications for conditions that were outside the scope of practice of dentistry.

- The dentist prescribed medications for herself/himself that were outside the practice of dentistry.

- Signing prescription blanks in advance of prescribing controlled substances.

**Box 4**
**Cases involving controlled substance in dentistry**

Source: David A. Keith email, January 29, 2020.

*I. Drug Enforcement Administration (DEA) action, documentation, prescribing for relative, lack of required training.* Specifically, Illinois Department of Financial and Professional Regulation alleged that Respondent prescribed Vicodin and Tramadol, on a monthly basis between 1996 and 2018, to treat a patient with temporomandibular joint dysfunction ("TMJ") syndrome, and failed to obtain ongoing diagnostic and/or radiological studies to verify and confirm the extent of that patient's continued TMJ symptoms, as well as authorizing numerous prescriptions for controlled substances without properly evaluating and monitoring the patient for signs and symptoms of drug addiction or abuse.

The stipulations in the Consent Order also included allegations that DEA Diversion Investigators (DIs) conducted an inspection of Respondent's dental practice and discovered that he prescribed Ambien and Codeine to his wife without documenting the prescriptions or dental examination necessary for those prescriptions in her chart. Id. at 2. He also stipulated that the DIs conducted a count of controlled substances and found a substantial amount of substances unaccounted for, including a shortage of 1034 Hydrocodone 5/500-mg tablets, a shortage of 500 tablets Hydrocodone 5/325 tablets, and a shortage of 1960 tablets Diazepam 5 mg. Id. In addition, according to the Consent Order, Respondent was unable to produce a biennial inventory, he failed to adequately maintain dispensing records for controlled substances, and he failed to maintain inventory records of controlled substances for 2 years. Id. The DIs also determined that (1) everyone in Respondent's dental office had access to the controlled substances cabinet; (b) Respondent kept a 500-count bottle of Vicodin, a 100-count bottle of Halcion, and a 500-count bottle of Valium in his home, a nonregistered address; and (c) Respondent kept a 100-count bottle of Vicodin in his desk drawer.

Respondent also failed to complete the required 9 hours of continuing education in sedation techniques for the 2009 to 2012 renewal cycle and failed to ensure that his staff had completed the requisite training to assist him in dental sedation procedures (https://www.deadiversion.usdoj.gov/fed_regs/actions/2019/fr0920_3.htm).

*II. Out-of-state case, practicing outside of the scope of practice.* A dentist prescribed Hydrocodone for his fiancée's father who had back pain. When this did not work, he prescribed Fentanyl patch 75 µg. The patient died within 24 hours of using the patch of a Fentanyl overdose because the patient was opiate naïve. Violations: treating a condition outside of scope of dental practice, treating an individual who was not a patient of record. Not understanding the potential risks of prescribing a strong opioid in an opiate-naïve individual. Hydrocodone has a 2.4 times higher mean morphine equivalency than Fentanyl patch (https://www.cdc.gov/drugoverdose/pdf/calculating_total_daily_dose-a.pdf).

Courtesy Karen Ryle MS RPh Associate Chief Pharmacist, Massachusetts General Hospital, Boston, MA- Email communication)

*III. Regulatory actions, multiple prescribing violations* (www.caewatch.org/board/dent/shankland/complaint.shtml). The dentist was charged with, among other complaints, prescribing excessive amounts of narcotic and sedative drugs. Specifically prescribing excessive amounts of opioids, prescribing meperidine chronically ("which is unequivocally contraindicated for chronic pain management"), prescribing 2 to 3 times the maximum daily dose of APAP (Acetaminophen) without any "periodic liver function tests to ensure that they are not experiencing hepatotoxicity," failing to "measure pain intensity and/or document your findings in order to assess benefits from opioids therapy," prescribing excessive amounts of carisoprodol and Ambien, prescribing opioids "chronically, without evidence of efforts to wean the patients' dosages or attempt alternative management of their condition." The dentist entered into a Consent Agreement with the State Board of Registration in Dentistry under which his dental license was suspended for 6 months, he agreed to complete 300 hours of continuing dental education with specific criteria, during 1 calendar year he was barred from prescribing any opioid narcotics or central nervous system–acting medications, and his records would be available for review and monitoring.

The State Board of Registration in Dentistry suspended the dentist's license to practice dentistry for 2 years. The specific issues were prescribing dosages and amounts of controlled substances that were not justified based on the diagnoses and conditions documented. The records reflected deficiencies, including lack of consistent intake history, few documented tests, lack of basis for diagnosis or rationale of treatment provided, lack of care coordination with primary care physicians and other specialists, lack of interval records documenting clinical progress, lack of documentation of discussion or use of alternative therapies and regular comprehensive examinations, and lack of exit strategies from treatment with controlled substances. The dentist failed to take appropriate action when the patients breached their opioid contracts and ignored signs of addiction to controlled substances, billed insurance companies for complicated follow-up visits without justification in the clinical record, and treated patients and prescribed medications for conditions that were outside the scope of practice of dentistry. He prescribed medications for himself that were outside the practice of dentistry. He signed prescription blanks in advance of prescribing controlled substances.

A brief review of the DEA Web site of cases that this agency brought against prescribers during 2004 to 2019 identifies approximately 20 involving dentists of a total of approximately about 600 registrant actions. The specific issues involved illegal distribution and trafficking of controlled substances, record-keeping violations. money laundering, prescribing opioids for sex, and involvement in a "pill mill." REF https://www.deadiversion,usdoj.gov>crim_admin_actions Accessed 1/6/2020.

*IV. Doctor shopping.* A 33-year-old female medical researcher complained of "jaw pain" and went to a local dentist. She had recently moved from a neighboring state and had no prior dental records or information available. Her previous medical history was noncontributory, and her dental examination revealed no pathology and mildly tender masseter muscles bilaterally. Home care measures and nonsteroidal inflammatory drugs as needed were recommended. The patient insisted that this would not control her pain and that she required Vicodin (hydrocodone), which had relieved her pain in the past. The dentist declined to prescribe an opioid as she felt that the patient's symptoms were out of proportion to her examination and that her symptoms could be adequately controlled by other means. She recommended referral to a specialist. A review of the patient's prescription drug monitory program (PDMP) revealed that in the past 6 months she had had 20 prescriptions: 16 for opioids and 2 for benzodiazepines. These had been issued by 18 prescribers, 15 of whom were identified as dentists practicing within a large metropolitan area within a few miles of each other. She had used 10 pharmacies. Her PDMP from the state in which she previously resided showed a similar pattern. This is an example of a knowledgeable individual who understood how dental practices work, recognizing that dentists, even within the same area were not likely to communicate on a regular basis. She was able to readily manipulate dentists to provide her with opioid prescriptions with little risk of discovery.

## ETHICAL OBLIGATIONS

The role of dentistry is expanding, and more attention is being paid to medical and psychiatric comorbidities that are commonly present among dental patients. The ADA and state dental societies have drawn attention to the importance of assessing substance use risk. Dental school curricula and state regulations are now requiring training in this area.[22] It is hoped that with this training we will see improved strategies for assessing the at-risk patient within general dental practice. Other articles in this issue review the background and importance of incorporating these approaches. **Box 5** includes the initial 2005 ADA Statement on Provision of Dental Treatment for Patients with Substance Use Disorders.

Vearrier discusses the ethical obligations of dentists when prescribing opioid medications in light of the ADA Principles of Ethics and Code of Professional Conduct.[23,24] Practitioners should be aware that some states have incorporated the ADA Principles

---

**Box 5**
**Statement on provision of dental treatment for patients with substance use disorders**

1. Dentists are urged to be aware of each patient's substance use history, and to take this into consideration when planning treatment and prescribing medications.

2. Dentists are encouraged to be knowledgeable about substance use disorders, both active and in remission, to safely prescribe controlled substances and other medications to patients with these disorders.

3. Dentists should draw on their professional judgment in advising patients who are heavy drinkers to cut back, or the users of illegal drugs to stop.

4. Dentists may want to be familiar with their community's treatment resources for patients with substance use disorders and be able to make referrals when indicated.

5. Dentists are encouraged to seek consultation with the patient's physician, when the patient has a history of alcoholism or other substance use disorder.

6. Dentists are urged to be current in their knowledge of pharmacology, including content related to drugs of abuse; recognition of contraindications to the delivery of epinephrine-containing local anesthetics; safe prescribing practices for patients with substance use disorders, both active and in remission; and management of patient emergencies that may result from unforeseen drug interactions.

7. Dentists are obliged to protect patient confidentiality of substance abuse treatment information, in accordance with applicable state and federal law.

*Adapted from* American Dental Association. Statement on the use of opioids in the treatment of dental pain. Available at: https://www.ada.org/en/advocacy/current-policies/substance-use-disorders. Copyright © 2005 American Dental Association. All rights reserved. Reprinted with permission.

---

of Ethics and Code of Professional Conduct into their regulations. Dentists have an obligation to keep up to date on advances in pain management so that they "do no harm" (Principle of Nonmaleficence). Dentists may be asked by patients to prescribe a controlled substance that is not indicated. Bearing in mind the Principle of Patient Autonomy (self-governance), the dentist has no obligation to comply with treatment requests that are not clinically indicated. Consistent with the interactive model based on communication, cooperation, and shared decision making, the dentist should inform the patient of the proposed treatment and any reasonable alternatives. Excessive or inappropriate requests by patients for opioids and other controlled substances may lead the dentist to suspect opioid misuse or abuse. Dentists have a duty to prescribe appropriately, protect the patient from harm, and refer the patient to a specialist if "doctor shopping" or diversion is suspected.[24]

## SUMMARY

Dentistry should be proud of its long history of providing responsible pain relief, as well as becoming more cautious in prescribing opioid medications when other safer pharmacologic options exist. Our fundamental training directs us to first eliminate the source of dental pain and prescribe analgesics only as adjunctive relief. Long before the recent opioid prescribing laws were enacted in various states, dentists have historically and appropriately been prescribing limited 2-day to 3-day supplies of opioids for acute severe postoperative dental pain (less than one-half the quantities now allowed by law in some states). It appears the United States is making progress in combating prescription opioid abuse,[17] but should efforts to limit diversion, abuse, and addiction fall short, prescribers may lose their abilities to prescribe some of these medications, thus limiting their options in providing effective pain management.[13] For a prescription to be valid, whether for controlled or noncontrolled medication, it must be written for a legitimate dental purpose and for a patient of record. Through self-regulation, the dental profession must continue to establish pain management guidelines based on scientific evidence and clinical experience to avoid further regulatory action restricting our prescribing privileges, which remain one of our most powerful therapeutic tools.

## FUNDING

Portions of this work were supported by the Educational and Research Foundation, Department of Oral and Maxillofacial Surgery, Massachusetts General Hospital, Boston, Massachusettsg. Partial support was received for the preparation of this article through a grant from "The Coverys Community Healthcare Foundation".

## DISCLOSURE

The authors have nothing to disclose.

## REFERENCES

1. Denisco RC, Kenna GA, O'Neil MG, et al. Prevention of prescription opioid abuse: the role of the dentist. J Am Dent Assoc 2011;142(7):800–10.
2. American Dental Association announces new policy to combat opioid epidemic. 2018. Available at: https://www.ada.org/en/press-room/news-releases/2018-archives/march/american-dental-association-announces-new-policy-to-combat-opioid-epidemic. Accessed January 28, 2020.
3. Commissioner of the FDA. History Milestones. U.S. Food and Drug Administration. Available at: https://www.fda.gov/about-fda/fdas-evolving-regulatory-powers/milestones-us-food-and-drug-law-history. Accessed January 27, 2020.
4. Thornhill MH, Suda KJ, Durkin MJ, et al. Is it time US dentistry ended its opioid dependence? J Am Dent Assoc 2019;150(10):883–9.
5. Harold RS. Prescription writing for dentists: ethical and legal guidelines. J Mass Dent Soc 2012;60(4):28–31.
6. Substance use disorders. Available at: https://www.ada.org/en/advocacy/current-policies/substance-use-disorders. Accessed January 27, 2020.
7. CDC guideline for prescribing opioids for chronic pain. Centers for Disease Control and Prevention. 2019. Available at: https://www.cdc.gov/drugoverdose/prescribing/guideline.html. Accessed January 29, 2020.
8. Opioid prescribing by dentists. Available at: https://www.ada.org/~/media/ADA/Science and Research/HPI/Files/HPIGraphic_0118_1.pdf?la=en. Accessed January 27, 2020.
9. Volkow ND. Characteristics of opioid prescriptions in 2009. JAMA 2011;305(13): 1299.
10. Tufts Health Care Institute. Executive summary: the role of dentists in preventing opioid abuse—Tufts Health Care Institute Program on Opioid Risk Management 12th Summit Meeting. Boston, March 11–12, 2010. Available at: www.thci.org/opioid/mar10docs/executivesummary.pdf. Accessed January 27, 2020.
11. Electronic prescribing of controlled substances: an overview. DrFirst. Available at: https://www.drfirst.com/products/epcs-gold/what-is-epcs/. Accessed January 29, 2020.

12. Electronic Prescribing of Controlled Substances (EPCS). Health IT guides. 2016. Available at: https://www.aafp.org/practice-management/health-it/epcs.html. Accessed January 29, 2020.
13. Registration support. DEA diversion control division. Available at: http://www.deadiversion.usdoj.gov/ecomm/e_rx/faq/faq.htm. Accessed January 29, 2020.
14. Larance B, Degenhardt L, Lintzeris N, et al. Definitions related to the use of pharmaceutical opioids: extramedical use, diversion, non-adherence and aberrant medication-related behaviors. Drug Alcohol Rev 2011;30(3):236–45.
15. ONeil M. The ADA practical guide to substance use disorders and safe prescribing. Hoboken (NJ): John Wiley and Sons Inc.; 2015.
16. Keith DA, Shannon TA, Kulich R. The prescription monitoring program data. What it can tell you. J Am Dent Assoc 2018;149(4):266–72.
17. The PDMP Training and Technical Assistance Center. The PDMP training and technical assistance center. Available at: http://www.pdmpassist.org/. Accessed January 27, 2020.
18. Dental guideline on prescribing opioids for acute pain management. 2017. Available at: http://www.breecollaborative.org/wp-content/uploads/Dental-Opioid-Recommendations-Final-2017.pdf. Accessed January 27, 2020.
19. Section 18. General Law - Part I, Title XV, Chapter 94C, Section 18. Available at: https://malegislature.gov/Laws/GeneralLaws/PartI/TitleXV/Chapter94c/Section18. Accessed January 28, 2020.
20. Armstrong D, Armstrong D, Orr M, et al. This dentist broke his opioid habit. Can the dental profession do the same? STAT. 2017. Available at: https://www.statnews.com/2017/02/14/dentists-opioid-prescribing/. Accessed January 27, 2020.
21. Dentists cases - Drug Enforcement Administration - DEA Search Results. Available at: www.deadiversion,usdoj.gov>crim_admin_actions. Accessed January 27, 2020.
22. Bennet J, Contreras OA, Stewart D. Dental schools addiction education regional summit proceedings. Available at: https://www.adea.org/uploadedfiles/adea/content_conversion_final/policy_advocacy/dental-schools-addiction-education-regional-summit-proceeding.pdf. Accessed January 27, 2020.
23. The ADA principles of ethics and code of conduct. ADA principles of ethics and code of professional conduct. Available at: https://www.ada.org/en/about-the-ada/principles-of-ethics-code-of-professional-conduct. Accessed January 27, 2020.
24. Vearrier L. What are the ethical considerations when prescribing patients opioid medications for acute dental pain? J Am Dent Assoc 2019;150(5):396–7.

Printed and bound by CPI Group (UK) Ltd, Croydon, CR0 4YY

03/10/2024

01040479-0011